CARE FREE KETO

HOW TO LOSE WEIGHT
AND HAVE FUN DOING IT!

IRICK WIGGINS

Table of Contents

PART 4 WHAT TO EAT 60

Meals 85

INTRODUCTION

What is CARE FREE KETO

Did you know that most overweight people will go on a diet and lose a significant amount of weight at least once in their life? However, studies show that 95% of them will gain all of it back within a few years. That's right, only 5% of people who lose weight are able to keep it off. This is because many people start diets with the idea that they are going to be really strict for a few months, lose the weight and eventually go back to eating whatever they want. This mindset is the problem. Luckily I was able to avoid that mindset and discover a much more sustainable one, a "Care-Free" approach to keto.

Care Free Keto is about getting healthy and staying healthy without the unnecessary struggle that comes with dieting. Starting with who you are today, and slowly turning into someone who CAN stick to a healthy lifestyle. Not through will-power or self-discipline but through building small habits that turn into big changes over time. And not just changes to your weight but changes to who you are, inside and out!

And the most important part of Care Free keto is that you get to do all of this while HAVING FUN! Because if you want to keep the weight off and continue to improve your health, you won't get there by picking a diet that makes you miserable. The food has to taste good. And the truth is you can still experience A LOT of mouth pleasure, avoid being stressed out 24/7 and blossom into your best self while living a keto lifestyle.

That being said, I am not here to tell you that Keto is the only way to lose weight and keep it off. Nor am I here to claim that potatoes are somehow responsible for the obesity pandemic. Keto was simply the lifestyle that helped me lose 80 lbs without having to focus on calories or anything else. And I just happened to fall in love with all of the other benefits it had to offer. So whether you plan to do keto for the rest of your life like me, or use it to kick-start your weight loss journey and then transition to a different lifestyle, you totally can. Because once you learn the principles of CARE FREE KETO you can apply them to anything!

PART 1
KETO BASICS

Chapter 1 : What You Need To Know

Before getting into the rest of the book, let's go over the keto basics and what you need to do in order to thrive on your keto journey! Keep in mind that many of these guidelines are not necessary when you're first starting out. The purpose of this book, as you will read in the following chapters, is to tell you my story and show you how to baby step your way to success.

What is keto?

Eating mostly fat, protein & fiber while cutting out the sugar and starchy carbs!

Keto is a way of eating where you limit the unnecessary carbs in your diet and focus on nutrient dense foods like quality meat, veggies, nuts, dairy & select fruits. The reduction in unnecessary carbs causes your body to stop depending on sugar for energy and start burning fat for fuel. A body that burns fat instead of sugar is in ketosis, and prolonged ketosis turns your body into a fat burning machine!

Examples of unnecessary carbs: Bread, sugar, rice, cereal, pasta, etc...

What isn't keto?

Getting most of your fat and protein from processed junk food

A lot of people assume keto is a diet that consists of processed meat, cream cheese & vegetable oil filled foods like mayonnaise. And while you technically can achieve a state of ketosis eating those foods, that is not what keto is about for most of the people who actually see success. The further you get away from "processed" foods and move towards whole foods, the healthier and more sustainable keto becomes.

This doesn't mean pepperoni slices, cream cheese & hellman's mayonnaise are totally off limits, it just means that you should center your meals around real food and use the other stuff to make it taste better. An example would be making chicken bacon ranch casserole. The primary ingredients are chicken, broccoli, bacon, & cheddar cheese but you also use ranch to add some flavor.

How many carbs can I have each day?

Total carb limit: 20-50g

This varies depending on the person eating the carbs and where the carbs are coming from, but the simple answer is somewhere between 20-50 total carbs per day. If the carbs are coming from high fiber things like sliced avocado, roasted broccoli & steamed cauliflower the number falls closer to 50. If the carbs are coming from foods that contain grains and sugar such as cereal or raisins the number falls around 20. Due to this variation, I find it much easier to simply focus on net carbs!

What are net carbs?

Net carbs are the only carbs you need to count

Net carbs are the only carbohydrates that your body is able to digest and use for energy. This means they are the only carbs that raise your blood sugar and have the ability to kick you out of ketosis.

How many net carbs can I have each day?

Net carb limit: 25g

In general 25g is the limit before your body stops burning fat and switches back to using carbs for energy. However, your limit may vary depending on activity level and the glycemic index of the carbs you are eating.

How do I count net carbs?

Total carbs - (fiber + sugar alcohol) = net carbs

total carbs - (fiber + sugar alcohol) = net carbs

To calculate net carbs you simply take the number of total carbs and subtract fiber and sugar alcohols from it. See examples below:

There is a new ingredient that you also want to subtract from total carbs and that ingredient is allulose! For some reason it isn't listed on the nutrition facts, so you will need to check the packaging to see if it is listed anywhere else. Most products that use allulose will give you a net carb calculation on the front or back and that is why the net carb count you calculate yourself might be

Nutrition Facts
4 servings per container
Serving size 0.5 cup(s) (120g)

Amount per serving
Calories **70**

% Daily Value*
Total Fat 3g — 4%
Saturated Fat 0g — 0%
Trans Fat 0g
Cholesterol 0mg — 0%
Sodium 140mg — 6%
Total Carbohydrate 9g — 3%
Dietary Fiber 3g — 11%
Total Sugars 4g
Includes 0g Added Sugars — 0%
Protein 3g

Vitamin D 0mcg — 0%
Calcium 41mg — 4%
Iron 1mg — 6%
Potassium 280mg — 6%

9g total carbohydrate - 3g dietary fiber = 6g net carbs

You do not subtract the sugars or added sugars, only sugar alcohol and fiber. Since there is no sugar alcohol on this label, you simply subtract fiber.

This product has 6 net carbs.

Nutrition Facts
Serving Size 1/2 cup (71g)
Servings Per Container 4

Amount Per Serving
Calories 150   Calories from Fat 120

% Daily Value*
Total Fat 14g — 22%
Saturated Fat 8g — 40%
Trans Fat 0g
Cholesterol 70mg — 23%
Sodium 15mg — 1%
Total Carbohydrate 10g — 3%
Dietary Fiber 2g — 8%
Sugars 0g
Sugar Alcohol 7g
Protein 2g

Vitamin A 8% • Vitamin C 0%
Calcium 4% • Iron 1%

10g total carbohydrate - 2g dietary fiber - 7g sugar alcohol = 1g net carbs

You do not subtract the sugars or added sugars, only sugar alcohol and fiber.

This product has 1 net carb.

different from the net carb count they show on the front of the package!

So this is the new formula I would use:

Total carbs - (fiber + sugar alcohol + allulose) = net carbs

Why else is it better to focus on net carbs?

Regulating blood sugar

Another reason I find it so important to limit net carbs instead of total carbs, is due to the fact that the best sources of carbs are typically loaded with fiber. And unless you are one of the rare people who thrive on a carnivore diet, there is literally no benefit to limiting fiber intake. If anything it could be harmful!

For example: If my limit is 20g total carbs per day and I eat a large nutritious avocado for breakfast I won't be able to eat any more carbs for the rest of the day. Despite the fact that almost ALL of the carbs in the avocado are coming from fiber, which will have zero impact on my blood sugar. And if the avocado uses up all of my carbs for the day I would end up skipping the mineral dense leafy greens at lunch and the antioxidant rich blueberries for dessert. Which doesn't make sense when you would still be in ketosis either way!

Another example of why limiting total carbs isn't the best idea is due to the glucose dampening effect of fiber. Basically, whenever you consume fiber at the beginning of a meal, it actually lowers the increase in blood sugar you experience from the net carbs you eat. So cutting back on fiber because it's a "carb" can actually make it harder to stay in ketosis. Anyone with a blood sugar monitor can do this experiment for themselves! Start your day with a piece of toast and check your blood sugar an hour later, you will notice a pretty big spike. Now for the next day, start out by eating an avocado and then eat a piece of toast and you will see a much lower spike in blood sugar.

But aren't carbs necessary?

Not all of them!

The argument you may have heard from an anti-keto dietician is that when carbohydrates are consumed they are converted into glucose, which is the preferred fuel source of the body. But the truth is; not only does the body love burning ketones for energy, it also does a great job of converting things like protein into glucose through a process called gluconeogenesis. This process paired with the power of ketosis is all that your body needs to thrive and be as healthy as ever!

While lots of people can thrive on a diet high in healthy carbohydrates like fruit, root vegetables, rice & even whole grains in some cases, that is not the only way to thrive. Especially if you are insulin resistant and can't even use those carbs efficiently. The only carbs I would say are NECESSARY for most people are not the kind that turn into glucose, but rather fiber rich fruits and vegetables. These carbs can help cultivate a healthy gut microbiome, fill you up and make it easier to go to the bathroom!

Pro tip: Another extremely healthy source of carbs is fermented foods like sauerkraut, kimchi, and unflavored greek yogurt!

How much fat and protein can I eat?

As much as it takes to stay on track

When starting out, you should eat as much fat and protein as it takes to feel full! As you progress and get the hang of things you can focus on adjusting the amount of protein and fat you consume based on your goals. But when you first start your keto journey and are getting used to this new way of life, it's going to be VERY challenging to resist carbs. And the more you allow yourself to fill up on quality protein and fat, the easier it will be to overcome those carb cravings.

For example.. Any time I tried to diet and lose weight the biggest struggle I faced was going to bed hungry. I absolutely hated it and it drove me to the point of binge eating several times. However, I didn't have that problem on keto because if I felt hungry all I had to do was go eat something that didn't have carbs in it. I wasn't worried about calories or fat, I was just putting my trust in the keto lifestyle and it truly paid off for me!

Isn't too much protein a bad thing?

No! Too little protein is a bad thing

Some of the first studies ever done on keto were focused on using it as a tool to help children with epilepsy. In this instance, it was important for the patients to be in a deep state of ketosis. Which usually requires about 80% of your caloric intake to be from fat sources. Leaving 15% of your calories to come from protein and 5% from carbs.

However, the average person today who simply wants to enjoy the benefits of mild ketosis doesn't need to take such an extreme approach. Many people who are looking for weight loss, cognitive benefits or any of the other benefits of keto will still see amazing results with a higher protein approach to keto.

Why is too little protein a bad thing?

Protein is the most essential macronutrient

There are studies showing people who thrive on a diet low in carbs and studies showing people who thrive on a diet low in fat. But it is very hard to find examples of people thriving on a diet low in protein. While it might be overwhelming to also track your protein, if you can aim for 20-40g of protein per meal you will be setting yourself up for success in many ways. Don't think of it as a way to bulk up and put on muscle, think of it as an anti-aging drug. As we age our bodies become less efficient at producing and using protein, which can lead to a rapid decline in overall health if we don't consume enough.

Pro tip: While breakfast is not essential, starting your day with protein is very beneficial. I typically add collagen and a protein shake to my coffee every morning.

What else is so good about keto?

Better energy, improved health & so much more!

Aside from the weight loss benefits of becoming a fat burning machine; It's important to know that when ketones become your primary fuel source, you will have consistent energy regardless of how often you are eating. So while people on a high carb diet depend on their next meal for energy, people on Keto never have to worry about missing a meal because they can simply get that energy from their stored body fat.

There are also various health benefits to following a keto diet, especially one that cuts out processed foods. Do some research and you will be amazed!

Do I really need to be in Ketosis?

Yes and no!

Keto is a way of eating that puts you in ketosis, so technically yes. If you want to do keto then you should aim to be in ketosis most of the time. But the principles of Care Free Keto can be applied to any variation of healthy eating. As long as you are eating less junk and progressing towards your goals, you are succeeding.

How does ketosis cause weight-loss?

It reduces your appetite.

If your goal is simply to lose weight, Keto is a great choice due to its main side effect; appetite suppression. The reduced appetite people experience on Keto is what makes so much fat loss possible without feeling miserable or stressing over calories. This happens because when you are no longer getting blood sugar spikes from high carb meals followed by the inevitable crashes a few hours later, you are able to feel full throughout the day without constantly needing more food to bring your blood sugar back up.

On a ketogenic diet, you're also less likely to be deceived by the imbalance of hunger hormones that you can experience on a standard American diet rich in processed foods. For example; Real hunger is when your body is in need of fuel. Hormonal hunger is when the hormone known as ghrelin which produces feelings of satiety, is outweighed by the hormone leptin, which produces feelings of hunger.

So next time you get a craving for food despite the fact that you are not malnourished in any way shape or form, remind yourself "This is hormonal and it will pass". That reminder can actually be a great mantra to repeat when the cravings come. Seriously, mantras are one of my favorite ways to overcome cravings / impulsive urges! Simply sit and breathe for 1-3 minutes and feel the hunger while repeating "this feeling of hunger is hormonal and it will pass".

Lastly, natural sources of protein and fat are just harder to overeat. For example; it is much easier to eat 30 twizzlers over the course of a day than it is to eat 30 tbsp of butter or 4.5 lbs of chicken despite all 3 having the same amount of calories.

How do I know if I'm in ketosis?

Test, test, test!

Testing your ketones is the best way to find out whether you're actually in ketosis or if you're simply eating a diet lower in carbs.

Types of tests:

Urine strips - You can test your ketones with urine strips for the first few weeks, which are the cheapest and easiest option. But your body will eventually stop excreting ketones through the urine when it is fully utilizing your ketones.

Blood monitor - A blood ketone monitor is the most accurate way to test your ketones & the option I recommend. Not to be confused with a glucose monitor which only shows you your blood sugar levels. My favorite brands are BioCoach & Keto-Mojo.

Breathalyzer - Certain breath monitors can tell you if you're in ketosis or not with great accuracy, while others aren't as reliable. A great brand that you can trust is Biosense.

Some other signs that you're in ketosis:

1. Not feeling very hungry.

2. Consistent energy all day.

3. Less emotional highs and lows throughout the day.

4. Less carb cravings.

What if I slip up and eat carbs?

Don't stress, just get back on track!

You might be wondering, what will happen if I go out for a non-keto dinner or wind up at a party and eat some carbs?

This is what to expect: Depending on how many carbs you had and how fat-adapted you are, it could take anywhere from 1-7 days to get back into ketosis. Which is totally fine because there is NO RUSH to get back into ketosis. The idea that you have to spend 24/7/365 in ketosis in order to see results is just not true. Any lifestyle that promotes eating less junk food over a long period of time will change your body so much that you could never undo it in one day, one weekend or even one vacation!

Here's what to do: Simply go back to 25g carbs per day! It's that simple. Doing some high intensity exercise can also help deplete the stored glycogen in your body & get you back to burning ketones. And unless you already have a healthy relationship with fasting, I don't recommend using prolonged fasts to get back into ketosis because this can lead to disordered eating.

What is fat-adapted?

When the body learns to use fat as its main source of energy

Becoming fat-adapted should be the main goal of anyone living a keto lifestyle. It is when your body prefers fat for energy opposed to carbs. You can typically expect to become fat-adapted within 60 days of being in ketosis. The only problem is that large slip ups can prolong the time it takes to become fat-adapted, making the process a bit more complex. So a simplified goal to guarantee you become fat-adapted would be:

2 months of 25g net carbs or less per day with ZERO slip ups.

However, it's important to know that there isn't a FAT-ADAPTED test you can take. And some people may become fat-adapted faster than others.

Pro Tip: If you accidentally eat 27g or 32g net carbs a few times during the 2 months you should be fine. But the higher that number goes, the more likely it is you will have to restart the 2 months.

How often can I cheat after becoming fat-adapted?

It depends on the person

Ideally you want to cheat as little as possible because even if you are fat-adapted it can do some serious damage to have several servings of Mac N Cheese and Ice Cream every week. However, if you're very active and have a healthy relationship with food, there is nothing wrong with a weekly serving of sweet potato fries or rice. Many people take this approach and have great success on a Cyclical Ketogenic Diet.

What about special occasions?

Enjoy yourself when the time is right

The truth about cheating is that you shouldn't even have to use the word cheating. We may go off-plan for a day or a meal, and that is totally fine. Or maybe we have holiday's that lead to a few days off-plan and that can be totally fine too!

For example: if I spend my anniversary at an all-inclusive resort, I am going to eat carbs for the 3-5 days I am there! I don't consider it cheating because it is a special occasion. You just want to be sure that these several day carb fests aren't happening more than a few times a year.

The only time I would advise against going off plan is if you are the type of person who will beat themselves up for not staying on track to the point where you don't even enjoy the special occasion anymore. Because at that point you aren't even enjoying yourself.

PART 2
MY STORY

Chapter 2 : Where It All Started

If you're anything like me, I bet you believe that diets don't work for you. Probably because they never have worked for you and even if they did, I bet the success was short-lived only for you to return to your previous weight or higher. So I don't blame you for having this belief. I bet you also feel like you are the type of person who lacks will-power around food. Meaning that if you even think about a Kit-Kat bar you have to have it. And "depriving" yourself of it stresses you out so much that you end up wanting TWO Kit-Kat bars! You probably can't even wind down at the end of the day unless you eat something sweet. Don't beat yourself up, I'm the same way.

I still identify as someone who has very little will-power around food. I still need (keto) sweets after dinner and I still allow myself the option to eat 37 servings of something if I'm hungry enough for it. Now you might be wondering "If you have such little control over your food choices, how are you doing keto?! And how are you at a healthy weight?". It's because slowly cutting out junk food and getting to the point where most of my meals consisted of healthy food, changed the relationship I had with food on a psychological and hormonal level. That is what allows me to feel totally satisfied after eating a steak for dinner and a keto ice cream bar for dessert without fighting the urge to get seconds or thirds. That is how I am able to live a Care Free lifestyle!

Let's go all the way back to childhood. This is where my unhealthy relationship with food began and I started putting on the pounds, as you can see below.

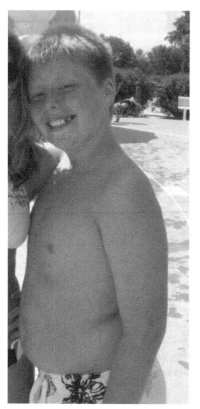

All of my life junk food was my happy place, no matter what was going on I could always count on it to make me happy. Whether it was pop-tarts for breakfast, mini corn dogs with spongebob Mac & Cheese for lunch or Wendy's fries dipped in a chocolate frosty for dinner. I've always been obsessed with the mouth pleasure that food is able to give me. The key word here is "pleasure".

Pleasure is something that we all want more of. No matter how happy we already feel, if we are offered the opportunity to receive more pleasure it's unlikely that we will say no. Just watch what happens when someone brings donuts to the break room at work! And when you look at how pleasurable the food in America has become over the past 50 years it's no surprise that almost everyone is fat. Things like baked chicken thighs, roasted potatoes and fresh fruit aren't that pleasurable compared to fried chicken dipped in BBQ sauce, french fries cooked in vegetable oil and candy that is literally designed to bombard the pleasure centers of your brain!

Now let's get back to how this rant about pleasure relates to my story. Growing up I was diagnosed with ADHD, which from the average person's point of view means that I had trouble sitting still and focusing in school. That is partially correct but there is a lot more to it than that, because what kid does want to sit still and focus on math? Based on conversations with doctors and the research I've done, ADHD can also mean this; It takes a lot of excitement to stimulate a person with ADHD. Which means they are often driven to pursue highly pleasurable experiences such as eating cookies to feel the same sense of stimulation another person would get from ordinary life.

The scientific reasoning behind this is due to a lack of dopamine receptors in the ADHD brain. Dopamine is the force that drives all action in humans. Without dopamine, you wouldn't even have enough motivation to stand up and get a drink of water, even if you were dying of thirst. It's that important. So if dopamine is the driving force that enables one to clean their room or do the dishes, what happens when someone doesn't have enough dopamine receptors? They are more likely to be driven towards things that produce big spikes in dopamine such as eating a box of cookies or playing a video game for several hours.

So while one person will experience an increase in dopamine from cleaning their room, a person with ADHD needs to anticipate a much greater reward for the same feeling. Replace cookies with drugs, alcohol or sex and it explains why the lack of impulse control that is so prevalent in people with ADHD can get you into serious trouble!

Considering what was going on in my brain paired with the easy access to junk food, my future was not looking bright. Because even people with normal impulse control are almost destined for weight gain and poor health in this environment. The infiltration of junk food into our diets over the past 50 years has created a literal pandemic of obesity. The problem with normalizing junk food is that food is meant to nourish us. It is meant to energize us and provide us with the nutrients we need to live a healthy life. And not only does junk food lack nutrients, it can deplete the nutrients we do have! Things like sugar and refined carbohydrates may provide calories but they do not provide nutrition. And when you grow up eating this stuff like we all probably did, your taste preferences, hormones and brain are being programmed to want more of it. To NEED more of it.

Sure, I had some healthy home-cooked dinners growing up but what about the rest of the day? Nobody told my parents not to give me Cheerios for breakfast or fruit juice with my turkey sandwich at lunch. In fact, my parents along with everybody else were encouraged to give us these things because they were "healthy" ... At the time I didn't demand to be served a grass fed ribeye and roasted carrots for dinner. I just asked for more candy and more fast food! Because after all, what makes a kid happier than sugar?

Aside from the frequent access I had to this stuff, a lot of my core memories were also accompanied by junk food which made it even harder to develop a healthy relationship with food. For example; If we went on a school trip they would give us happy meals!

If we went to an amusement park we got ice cream and pizza! Essentially ALL of my happy memories growing up were accompanied by it in one way or another. Even today, 20 years later, many of my happy memories are made around the dinner table or at all-inclusive resorts. This means that I don't just see orange chicken and crab rangoon as a yummy and pleasurable meal, it's also symbolic of the times my friends and I would spend hours upon hours at the mall blowing our Christmas money on cool T-shirts and Nike socks.

A lot of the kids I grew up with in this environment didn't start putting on weight until later in life. Although the statistics are now starting to show that more and more kids are becoming overweight as the junk food craze worsens. Yes... it's getting worse! But at the time I was one of the unlucky ones who did get fat and it was an emotional roller coaster.

Chapter 3: The Chubby Kid

The first memory of my weight being a problem is from third grade. Our little league football team was pretty competitive and all I wanted to do was make tackles and score touchdowns. The problem was that I was too short and weak to be a lineman and too chubby and slow to be anything else. So my position was THE BENCH. To make things worse, our team went undefeated and made it all the way to the championship that year. Which should have been exciting. But I didn't play a single minute in that game and I remember feeling like the biggest loser in the world.

Another memory that still haunts me is from 7th grade. This was probably my emotional rock bottom. After another year of riding the bench in football, one of my best friends encouraged me to try wrestling. I thought this was my chance to finally be good at something. Boy was I wrong. Being 40 pounds overweight I was put in the same weight class as the 8th graders who had already gone through puberty. Meaning these kids were 150 lbs of muscle while I was 150 lbs of fat. My record that year was 0-11. That's right, zero wins and eleven losses. I couldn't have felt more defeated, literally and emotionally.

Not being good at sports might seem like it's not a big deal to most people, as it really isn't in the grand scheme of things. But when you grow up in Ohio where there is literally nothing to do, sports are everything. My hometown treated every high school football game like the Super Bowl. So not only was my level of athleticism the only path to validation from adults, it was the only thing that mattered for determining my spot in the social hierarchy. That meant all of my friends got to date whoever they wanted, while I was sent straight to the friendzone. It meant that all of the teachers and coaches treated my friends like royalty while I was viewed as the kid who just tagged along and caused trouble.

After my 0-11 record in wrestling it felt like my only option in climbing up the social ladder was to embrace being the chubby kid and use self deprecation to make people laugh. Which further solidified my spot as the trouble maker because making teenagers laugh is not an easy job and breaking the rules is often a necessary means. At this point any sense of self worth I had left was long gone. And while I did gain acceptance from the "cool" kids, it never felt real because I knew deep down I wasn't one of them. But that didn't stop me from chasing their acceptance, which meant I was also extremely susceptible to peer pressure. Whether they were telling me to have a basement boxing match with the older and stronger kid only to get knocked out or challenging me to chug a can of beer, I didn't hesitate once.

And if all of this pressure to fit in wasn't enough of a problem, I still had the dark cloud of my body image hanging over me. I remember stretching out my shirts so they didn't highlight my man boobs & stomach, hunching over when I sat down so people wouldn't look at my body and even crying myself to sleep because I couldn't get a girlfriend. I also remember becoming a pro at taking flip-phone mirror selfies from the perfect angles to make myself appear thinner on my Myspace profile. But as soon as we took group photos for the school dance that year, the facade came crumbling down.

Going into high school was another difficult time for me. Because as previously discussed, I was the poster-child for giving in to peer pressure. And while the friends I had in my age group were still playing outside and being kids, I was focused on gaining acceptance from the older kids. Which meant I was not playing outside and being a kid anymore. The first 2 years of highschool are kind of a blur to me because they were spent smoking pot, trying to find parties & doing whatever it took for the older kids to keep me around. But I do know that my weight would fluctuate wildly, as I would go on diets in hopes of joining the wrestling team only to binge on taco bell, gain it all back and quit before the season even started.

Seeing these fluctuations in my weight gave me the hope that if I just made the right lifestyle changes, I could get my life on track and be known for something more than the kid who makes everyone laugh. It felt like I still had a chance to get in shape and become the breakout star that our football team needed or make it to the state tournament in wrestling. I remember trying to go for runs. I could also have used the number 4 instead of the word, because I probably went on 4 runs total. I remember trying to eat low fat, and while that worked for a few months, I eventually fell back into my old eating habits.

Chapter 4: Major Changes

Then when I was 17 something happened that changed the entire course of my life. My friends and I took a spring break trip to Panama City Beach, FL. which was about a 12 hour drive from where we lived in Ohio. In order to save money we booked one room for 6 of us. Which as you can imagine was a nightmare. But aside from being crammed in the room it actually was a fun trip. We did all of the mischievous things that teenagers do and by the end of the trip we were sleep deprived, hungover and not equipped to drive home. To make things worse we had the bright idea of leaving the night before check-out. That way we wouldn't have to spend our last day of spring break sitting in the car. So we left in the middle of the night on zero sleep.

All I remember after that is being pulled out of a car on the side of the road by some people who stopped to help us. Apparently my friend had fallen asleep behind the wheel and the car flipped, slid upside down on the highway and eventually went into a ditch. I was not wearing a seatbelt and while the car was sliding upside down on the road I was against the back windshield. At least that was the only way they could explain how I had roadrash, as a lot of skin on my back and shoulder got ripped off. Luckily I was the only person with any serious injuries and surprisingly enough, I didn't even feel any pain. All I could think about was how thankful I was to be alive. It was the strangest experience because while everyone else was freaking out and worried, I just felt like a higher power had saved me and knew everything was going to be okay.

Having a near death experience is probably the best thing that ever happened to me because it instantly gave me a sense of purpose. It showed me how ridiculous it was that I had spent the past 7 years chasing acceptance and trying to fit in rather than being who I truly wanted to be. It also showed me that I was here for a reason and while I didn't know exactly what that reason was, it was the first time where I felt like my life mattered. After returning home I got showered with love and support from everyone in our small town which was a really good feeling, but as you can probably guess I also got showered with sugary desserts and treats.

That was actually how I got into the habit of consuming sugary drinks. I grew up as someone who loved water and didn't really care for anything else. But one of the get-well-soon gifts that I received was a big jug of my friend's Dad's famous sweet tea. Which had double the sugar of regular sweet tea. And I was starting my day with it, drinking it with every meal and having it before bed too. Eventually I ran out, and you know what happened? They brought me more!! But this time it was 2 jugs. Eventually I started making my own and before I knew it I was hooked.

Other than the fact that sugary drinks are adding hundreds of unnecessary calories to your daily intake, there is another problem to address. Consuming sugar by itself like this will send your blood sugar to the moon and set you up for overeating and cravings all day. Sugary drinks like fruit juice and soda are totally different from foods that naturally have sugar. For example, the sugar in most fruit is intertwined with fiber and that will slow the rate at which your body absorbs it, which prevents a huge spike in blood glucose. Even having a sugary sauce on your chicken and broccoli isn't totally detrimental because the fat, protein and fiber from your meal is slowing your glucose response too. But eat that sauce by itself and you are doomed.

Aside from my new found love of sugary drinks, this was still a monumental time for me because I finally started piecing my life together and became clear about the future I wanted for myself. At the time I wanted to become a music producer and rapper, which might seem silly but I was dead serious about becoming the next big thing despite having zero talent. That delusional ambition helped me in a lot of ways though because I no longer cared about fitting in with the cool kids and I also realized that alcohol was not for me. It was the first time in my life where I felt like my own person with my own goals. But now that I wasn't going out and partying anymore, I turned to food in a way like never before. It was my new fix.

The small town I grew up in only had a handful of restaurants and my favorite was Dairy Queen. Sometimes I would get 2 blizzards a day because just 1 couldn't satisfy me. Not to mention how good those chicken baskets were. I was still using marijuana though as most aspiring rappers do, which is where I tried placing the blame for my poor eating habits. Even though plenty of my friends who also had the munchies didn't join me on my second trip to Dairy Queen. The fact that I was the only one who needed 2 blizzards to feel satisfied caused me to start feeling like things were different for me and I wondered if something was wrong with me. I didn't understand why I wasn't satisfied with 1 serving at dinner, or why the list of candy I asked my dad for on his way home from work every day looked like a grocery list.

Fast forward a year or two and I was no longer using marijuana which meant I didn't have the munchies anymore, but even without them I was still craving junk food all day. This is actually when I ballooned up to my highest weight of 240 lbs. Reflecting on this experience, I can see what the problem really was. I had the tendency to quickly develop an addictive relationship to anything that brought me pleasure. So everytime I cut out a bad habit like drinking or smoking pot I simply replaced it with food.

This is actually a common occurrence, just go to an AA meeting and you will find many people who replaced their alcohol use with cigarettes, coffee, food or all three! But at the time I was 19 years old and I simply wasn't aware enough to realize that this was the force driving my food addiction. All I knew was that if I ever wanted to feel comfortable in my body I would have to change something, but it felt so out of reach because I just didn't believe that I could. Even after discovering the power of positive thinking and realizing that I was in charge of the way I experienced life, I simply couldn't make any healthy habits stick.

Chapter 5: Starting Small

This is where taking baby steps towards a healthy lifestyle saved me.

Despite being in this unhealthy relationship with food and holding on to the belief that I couldn't change it, I was still somewhat optimistic about my ability to reach other life goals. That optimism inspired me to start watching self-help videos on youtube and reading self-help books. In 2015 I eventually stumbled upon a piece of advice that really made things click into place for me. I was working midnights at a Kohl's warehouse, listening to an audiobook on meditation and the author said "If you can't meditate for 20 minutes a day, start with 3 minutes a day" which kind of opened my mind to the idea of baby steps. I immediately started meditating for 3 minutes a day, which turned into 5 and eventually turned into 20.

That was the first time I had ever been consistent with anything in my life. And that feeling of consistency was the first step towards shifting my entire identity over the next few years. I was no longer the type of person who fantasized about meditating or the type of person who told myself I'll start tomorrow, I was the type of person who wanted to start meditating every day and actually did it. Reflecting on this experience I am still in awe at how incredible it is that committing to something as simple as sitting still for 3 minutes a day opened the door to an entirely new life for me.

After a few months of meditating daily I was totally obsessed with this new found power in taking baby steps. It felt like I finally knew the secret to accomplish anything in life. So I decided to take a similar approach towards fixing my eating habits. I started with a small step that I knew I could realistically stick to. I simply started adding healthy foods to the food I was already eating. That helped me stop believing I was the type of person who had no control over my eating habits and start identifying as someone who CAN make healthy choices. This identity shift was crucial for the next phase of my life.

If there is one piece of advice I would give to someone who is struggling with their eating habits, it's to look up the benefits of the healthy foods that you enjoy eating. Then simply start out by adding those things to your meals. It gets you excited about eating the good stuff and it gives you a feeling of empowerment because you start to believe that you do have some control over your eating habits. Which is crucial because if you don't believe that you can change, you probably won't.

So instead of looking up how terrible ice cream was for me, I looked up the benefits of blueberries and avocados. This caused me to add more blueberries to my milkshakes, which naturally caused me to use less ice cream. Then I tried adding avocados and peanut butter to them as well. It was actually pretty good and I didn't feel restricted at all. Before I knew it I was eating salads every day and my milkshakes had turned into smoothies. I still wasn't experiencing much weight loss but I did feel better. I didn't realize it at the time but all of these small changes to my habits were preparing me to make the jump into a low carb lifestyle.

Chapter 6: Discovering Keto

Finally in 2016 I was listening to a podcast where I learned about the Keto / Low Carb Lifestyle and decided to give it a try. The reason I felt like this diet was different from the others and actually could be the one for me is because it didn't involve calorie counting as the main focus. Which was the most important part in giving me the confidence to try it. This was the first time I felt like I could succeed on my weight loss journey because the number one reason I failed at everything else was due to my inability to stop myself from eating if I felt hungry. I've always thought the idea that people are able to stop eating despite still being hungry was insane. Even today after changing my views on calorie counting and understanding that it can be implemented in a healthy way, I still don't see a calorie limit being enough motivation for me to hit the brakes on food if I'm truly hungry.

It wasn't an easy journey at the beginning, but the fact that I never had to make myself feel hungry was a total game changer. If I was still hungry after dinner, I would go make another plate. If I was still hungry after my second plate, I would go make a third plate. And if I was still hungry after my third plate, I would make a fourth plate. This sense of freedom got me through the beginning stages of Keto without feeling the need to give up when it got really hard. And funny enough, I rarely had to make a second or third plate due to the fact that I was now eating satiating foods.

The problem with trying to lose weight on the Standard American Diet is that it's not satiating at all. If you start your day with processed carbs in the form of a bagel or a frappuccino you are setting yourself up for insatiable cravings all day. And if you do successfully resist them at lunch and dinner, the cravings will become unbearable at night. However, if you start your day with good sources of protein and fat such as eggs and an avocado you will send a signal to the hunger center of your brain that you are not starving and that you don't need to aggressively seek out high calorie foods.

An average day of eating for me during the first year was not perfect and I still had a lot to learn, but I was definitely dropping pounds and feeling much better. My go-to breakfast was usually eggs with some sauteed spinach or peppers and I would have a large salad for lunch. At the time I was still living with my parents, so for dinner I would get creative in ketofying whatever they had. If it was fast food I would get a burger without the bun.

If it was a salisbury steak, I would literally rinse off the sauce and eat it with my own vegetables instead of mashed potatoes. For dessert I would usually end up eating some strawberries and peanut butter. However, if I had enough carbs left for the day I would sometimes eat half a bowl of lucky charms with unsweetened almond milk. Which is not a good idea by the way.

The reason I say it's not a good idea to use up all of your carbs on highly processed grains and sugars such as lucky charms, skittles, etc.. is for two reasons. The first reason is because these foods are very high on the glycemic index, meaning they spike your blood sugar to much higher levels than other carbs. So eating 25g of high glycemic carbs all at once will immediately knock you out of ketosis. Whereas 20-30g of low glycemic carbs such as veggies and nuts will keep your blood sugar low and ketones high. The second reason it's not a great idea is because you typically want your carbs to be broken up into 2-3 meals over the course of an entire day. Especially if you are eating fun keto foods that are a bit higher on the glycemic index like low carb tortillas and bread. But in the case that you get most of your carbs from high fiber veggies and nuts it shouldn't be a problem to consume all of your carbs in one meal.

Aside from the occasional bowl of lucky charms, another major flaw in my approach to keto was including weekly cheat days. While they did not stop me from dropping an astonishing 60 lbs the first year. They did make it impossible to get fat adapted which meant I was constantly switching back and forth between carbs and fat as my primary source of energy in a very inefficient way. Refer to the section "KETO BASICS" for an explanation of the science behind this.

The main problem with my weekly cheat days though was in the way that I approached them. I didn't simply allow myself a cheat meal for dinner or have a calm and controlled day of higher carb foods that would still be considered healthy. No, there was none of that. Moderation was literally non-existent. I went on a mission to fit as much fast food into my stomach as humanly possible.

I recognize that this type of behavior especially if followed by guilt, shame and an unhealthy level of food restriction is a classic example of disordered eating. So if that is your experience with cheat days it is extremely important that you seek psychological help.

Here is how an average cheat day would go for me...

Thursday night at midnight I would begin eating the Subway sandwich, pint of ice cream and Kit-Kat that I bought in advance. Then I would wake up to a breakfast sandwich & Frappuccino. Lunch involved a trip to Taco Bell and McDonald's where I would first get a chicken Quesadilla to put in the refrigerator and eat later on. Because reheating fries is terrible but reheating a quesadilla is actually delicious! Then at McDonald's I would get the chicken nuggets or chicken tenders, a large fry & seven sides of sweet & sour. At the time they had the Buttermilk Crispy Chicken Tenders and I would use one cup of sweet and sour per chicken tender. That was usually eaten in the parking lot so the fries wouldn't get cold and the tenders would still be crispy. Dinner involved a trip to Pizza Hut and a final stop at United Dairy Farmers for a milkshake.

While I would never advocate for this behavior around food, the thing that separated my way of doing things from a full blown eating disorder was the fact that I didn't feel any guilt nor did I find it necessary to take extreme measures and dramatically cut back on food intake afterwards. I simply went back to my very non-restrictive keto lifestyle. I also feel that it would be unfair to blame keto for causing this. Because whatever "diet" I went on prior to keto involved cheat days AT LEAST once a week, but usually more than that. And if I wasn't on a diet the only thing stopping that from becoming my daily life was not being able to afford fast food 3x per day every day. Keto made it easier for me to resist these urges due to the satiating nature of all the fat and protein I was eating.

Immediately after a cheat day I would feel so stuffed that the idea of eating more fast-food gave me the ick and I couldn't wait to get back to salads with grilled chicken. That feeling didn't last long though because by Monday or Tuesday the cravings would eventually return. However, knowing that I just had to wait until Friday was helpful in resisting the urge to eat more junk. But if something stressful happened in the middle of the week, forget it, all will-power went out the window and I would start my cheat day early.

I remember one time I lost a really important document and spent so much time searching for it without any luck. I was so frustrated, it felt like I was going to go insane. Eventually the idea of escaping the frustration with a milkshake entered my mind and all of a sudden I was driving to get one. I remembered the moment I thought about the milkshake and the moment I was in the car on my way to McDonald's, but I couldn't remember anything in between. it was like I had instantly been possessed.

All of the negativity that was consuming me had been soothed with the promise of mouth pleasure. I was so excited for this milkshake and everything that would come along with it. After I ordered my usual meal with a large chocolate milkshake I started planning everything else I was going to eat. I went from highly stressed to totally excited and euphoric in an instant. The only way to describe that level of excitement is like imagining you're back in college and your crush asked you to come over at 12 AM. You know it's bad, but some primal urge within is flooding your brain with reward chemicals.

My second year started out pretty similar to the first year except I was learning more about what to eat and what to avoid, I was getting creative with recipes and I even started going for walks outside. I remember my first "keto creation" was a pizza on low carb pita bread. It was actually really delicious and became a staple in my diet. At the time I didn't know there were so many delicious keto recipes out there, so I kept my diet pretty simple and saved the excessive mouth pleasure for my cheat days.

The only problem during this time was that my weight was at a stand still for about 8 months. I loved how I felt and truly enjoyed this new lifestyle so I didn't give up on it, but I was pretty discouraged. I didn't even realize why I was stalling at first. Was I just meant to be overweight? Was I already at a healthy weight and struggling with body dysmorphia? A lot was going through my mind but I eventually considered the idea that if I had less cheat days I might have an easier time losing the last 20 pounds.

Giving up weekly cheats was extremely hard at first so instead of cutting them out completely I simply tried to have them every other week. To my surprise it wasn't so bad, if anything it actually got easier to resist carbs. I also noticed that my body was feeling better and my energy levels were consistently higher! All of this positive reinforcement inspired me to switch them to once per month. It got to a point where it wasn't even about weight loss anymore. Sure, I was still checking my progress on the scale but this new approach to keto felt like something I could sustain forever.

Chapter 7: Skinny Fat

Finally in March 2018, after a few months of this change and 2 full years of Keto I was able to get to my goal weight of 160 lbs. This was also around the time I started an Instagram page to share my keto journey. Looking back on it, it's funny how right before I reached my goal I started to fall in love with the lifestyle beyond a means for weight loss. It actually seems like that is the key to everything in life. If you only do something for the end goal and your heart isn't in it for the long term, it rarely works out. For example; When I was building KetoSnackz I wasn't focused on making money and becoming an influencer. I just wanted to help people on their weight loss journey. However, it eventually became my full time career and while I'm by no means rolling in the dough, I can afford to live comfortably doing what I love.

So I had finally hit my goal and while this accomplishment felt great at first, the feeling of victory eventually faded. Because no matter how toned you are as a woman or how large your arms are as a man there is always someone to compare yourself to who looks better. This is when my body dysmorphia really kicked in. I would see myself from certain angles and be like "ew I still look chubby". Or I would see myself from another angle and be like "ew now i'm just skinny-fat". I knew I was at a healthy weight but I still had a hard time looking at my body without cringing.

This went on for the next several months. It felt like my self esteem was in purgatory. While I felt great about my overall health and the lifestyle change I didn't feel confident about my body at all. The only reason I didn't try to lose more weight was because I simply didn't have the discipline to stop eating when I was still hungry. Plus, I knew that exercise for weight loss wasn't something I could stick to because everytime I went to the gym I would burn 200 calories and just feel guilty that I didn't burn more, which discouraged me from going the next day.

Towards the end of 2018 I got the idea that maybe lifting weights will give me the confidence I need. Instead of losing the "fat" that bothered me so much I figured that getting some muscle would make me feel good about myself. The problem was that I didn't feel comfortable enough to go lift weights at the gym because I was so scared everyone would judge me for doing it wrong or not lifting enough weight. But after some debating, I finally got the courage to take the first baby step and just use the elliptical. I knew that I had to start somewhere and at least on the elliptical I don't have to worry about being in anybody's way. It's funny how I thought that the weight loss would give me self esteem yet I still was worried about "being in people's way" at the gym, as if they were superior to me.

Eventually I decided to make the leap from elliptical to weights. While it was extremely uncomfortable and I didn't feel ready at all, I knew the time was never going to be right so I stopped making excuses and just did it. I started out by using one machine and then quickly going back to the elliptical. I still remember sitting on that chest press machine looking at all the other people with perfect bodies and feeling so ashamed of mine. I didn't let it stop me though and after a few trips to the gym I decided to try another machine. Before I knew it I was doing pull ups and chin ups as well. I started to look at other peoples bodies and feel inspired rather than ashamed. I think this change started to happen for a few reasons.

The first reason is that the more I stepped out of my comfort zone the better I felt about myself. Because it's one thing to overcome poor eating habits in the privacy of your home, but to try and undergo a fitness transformation in a public setting is rough. So if you are at a place where you hate the gym, I totally feel you. But just remember that the harder it is to overcome something the more confident you will feel after doing it. If getting your life on track was easy, everyone would do it and it wouldn't feel like an accomplishment.

The second reason is that I started listening to podcasts about health and fitness and I remember an episode where a body builder was telling his story about how he got started and I remember thinking... "Wow he was just like me at one point". It kind of changed the way I saw muscular people at the gym. Instead of thinking of them as these superior beings looking down on me, I started to think they are probably rooting for me because they know what it's like to be in my shoes.

The same applies to being an overweight woman at the gym. Most of the girls there weren't born with toned bodies and perfect butts. And the ones who may have been genetically gifted might only be 2 kids and 10 years of career stress away from being in your shoes. So instead of comparing yourself to them, recognize that you already are beautiful and then compare yourself to who you were the day before! Because that is what successful people do.

While I still didn't like the way my body looked I was able to find some happiness in going to the gym and making progress. I also realized that doing a hard workout requires a lot of effort and makes it nearly impossible to focus on what other people are doing. So if anyone reading this thinks that all of the super fit people at the gym are obsessing over you and judging your body, I've got some news for you; They're not. Maybe the beginners are looking at you but anyone who is actually doing a hard workout is focused on recovering between sets, not watching you do yours.

After a few months of lifting weights I started learning about the mental health benefits of exercise and that changed everything for me. While I was definitely enjoying my workouts more than when I started, I still wasn't in love with working out. I just saw it as a means to an end. But after learning about all of the mental health benefits beyond changing my body composition I knew this was the next step to change my life forever. It's not that I had these crippling bouts of depression or daily panic attacks, but I've always struggled with motivation and calming myself down during stressful situations. So to learn that exercise was a natural remedy to help with these things, it quickly became a habitual part of my life.

Imagine you have low levels of excitement for life and you're also struggling with anxiety, then someone comes along and offers you a pill that will make everything a little bit better. Wouldn't you take it? Well that pill is called exercise. I want to clarify that I am not anti-medication. Medication is one of the most powerful tools that can be used to heal us. I just believe that exercise should be given an equal amount of credit for its ability to heal us, or rather prevent us from needing to be healed in the first place. For example; If you've spent the majority of your life with a happiness level of 7 out of 10, and then for the past 2 years you've been at a 3 or 4, it might be wise to see a mental health professional and take the medication they prescribe you. But what would also be wise is to look at how your lifestyle has changed and see if there is more to the story.

Maybe the pandemic stopped you from working out and caused you to start over-eating lots of junk food. And even with the world opening back up, the extra 40 pounds you put on are eating away at your confidence and preventing you from going to the spin class you used to love. Don't you think that poor eating habits, sedentary lifestyle and lack of community are also contributing to your decline in happiness? Anyone with access to PubMed can spend 10 minutes finding numerous studies that show how all of these things are major factors in developing depression.

This isn't meant to diminish the many instances of people who are born with a chemical imbalance, in which lifestyle changes can help but may never offer a cure. It is simply explaining what might happen if the average person falls out of their healthy habits and as a result has lower levels of happiness. Because at the end of the day, serotonin is the main chemical responsible for happiness and contentment with one's life. And do you know what boosts serotonin? Positive lifestyle habits such as; Sunlight, exercise, healthy foods, human connection & stress management.

My theory is that these habits boost serotonin in two ways. The first is simply on a biological level. However, I also believe that the average person who is living a life they are not proud of will have a harder time making serotonin than someone who is creating a life that they feel good about. Because gratitude and even where you stand in your peer group can also have a major influence on serotonin levels. And it's much easier to be thankful for what you have and proud of where you are in life if you crushed your to-do list than if you spent all day eating hot cheetos.

The last thing I will say on this topic before moving on is I am aware that in a lot of cases the depression has gotten so bad you aren't able to undo these negative lifestyle changes without the help of medication. Taking advantage of mental health resources like medication, therapy, etc.. is something I wholeheartedly support and have done myself. But that doesn't mean the medication can replace the sense of purpose and happiness you will gain from becoming a person you are proud of being. So take the medication if the doctor prescribes it, but don't forget that the medication is meant to help you build a better life. And it will take something a lot stronger than antidepressants to feel "happy" about a life that is spent watching reality TV and eating oreos all day.

Chapter 8: Finding Happiness

So I had finally created the habit of working out and life was going great. My Instagram page even started to blow up which was extremely exciting. But in Spring of 2019 I injured my shoulder trying to lift too much weight without a spotter and I was so scared that all of this excitement I had built around going to the gym was going to disappear. The first thing I did was give up cheat days until I got better because I felt like my body would have a much harder time recovering if I was shoving a bunch of inflammatory junk into it. The next thing I did was try running.

My first run lasted for 11 minutes at a very slow pace. I didn't even run an entire mile. But I did notice that I felt really good for the rest of the day, even better than I felt after lifting weights. The next day I ran for about 12 minutes and actually made it a mile. On the third day the gym was closed because they were doing some remodeling so I went running at the nature park near my gym and made it an entire 20 minutes. There was something about running outside that felt totally different than running on a treadmill. Rather than being confined to a small rectangle, I felt free. I felt like I had total control of the experience. Pretty soon I was going on 8 mile runs and felt like I had finally found the happy pill I needed.

After this break from cheat days and my new found happiness in running, my life had reached an all time high! Sticking to keto felt pretty much effortless. My Instagram page went from a fun hobby to a potential career path. And my shoulder was finally better which meant I could lift weights again.

Despite how excited I was to get back into weight lifting, I quickly realized that I got way more happiness out of running. So I decided to cut back on lifting weights and put most of my effort into running. At first it was a tough decision to make because all of the health gurus I followed were saying to prioritize weight lifting and that if you are going to run you only need to do sprints once or twice a week, which I hated. But I slowly came to realize that it doesn't matter what the optimal fitness routine is unless you are a bodybuilder or someone who is really passionate about maximizing their fitness.

This mindset around exercise that emphasizes doing what you enjoy is especially important to embrace if you are at the beginning of your fitness journey or struggling to stay on track. Because by prioritizing the activity that you enjoy the most you will be much less likely to fall back into a sedentary lifestyle which is the real killer. The healthiest people are those who actually stick to the activity they set out to do and if you are more likely to walk 4 miles a day than lift weights 4x a week, keep on walking! The only caveat to this is that you should give everything a chance before you decide what you like. Because had I never injured my shoulder or had the gym never been closed that day forcing me to go for my run outside, I wouldn't have realized what my favorite activity was.

Another change that happened in my life while I started my running journey was that I decided to start answering questions through live-streams on Instagram. Despite having tons of followers, my live-streams consisted of around 100 people but some of those people became my closest friends. It was the first time I felt like I belonged somewhere. Gaining this sense of community was also a major contributor in not feeling the need to turn to food for happiness anymore. Because it turns out that little break from cheat days due to my shoulder injury would actually turn into 2 years of zero cheat days!

It was hard to believe that these daily hangouts with people on the same path as me gave me a greater sense of wholeness than I used to get from food. And this wholeness was long lasting which made it even better. So whether you have to go on an app like "Meetup" and find people with similar hobbies, reconnect with an old friend group or even go to Church... It can be extremely helpful to find some sort of connection with others. Because if food is the highlight of your day, every day, it might mean that you are traveling the world in search of the best cuisine out there but the more likely scenario is that your life is lacking in some areas. Especially if the food that makes you so happy is prepackaged junk.

The feedback I was getting from these daily hangouts also showed me how much I had learned about what people like me are struggling with and what we needed to succeed. So after answering the same questions over and over again my audience suggested I put everything in a book. To be honest, an author was never something that I saw myself as but the idea of putting all of this information in a book did make sense. Especially as a way to share all of the new recipes I had been working on.

At this point in my life I had no idea how to create a book. But after watching a few youtube videos and deciding to start no matter how unqualified I felt, I got it done. So in July of 2019 "Breaking up with Carbs" hit the shelves. Or rather came out on Amazon because that is the only place it was being sold. Shortly after I realized that it was sloppily put together and could have been much better so I connected with a friend who helped me edit a new and updated version. That version came out in February of 2020.

The book was received much better than the first version and my Instagram page was continuing to grow. After all of the messages and book reviews from people who used my advice to overcome obesity, my life's purpose became very clear: To help as many people get their health on track as I possibly can. Once I had this realization it also occurred to me that in order to really fulfill this purpose I had to get around other people who are using social media to promote a health focused message. And Ohio was NOT the place for that to happen. So on 3 weeks notice I decided to move out of my parents house and venture off on my own to Austin, TX.

Chapter 9: Hello Austin! and... Ana?

Being a content creator is a very financially insecure path because you never know where your next paycheck is coming from. And even if someone is offering you money, you can't always say yes because you don't want to promote products that you don't believe in. So this was a scary decision, especially during the height of the pandemic. But I had such a strong desire to chase my dream that I didn't care. I had to go for it. I didn't tour apartments, I didn't visit the city, I literally picked the first place I saw that had a kitchen island so I could make cooking videos. They had a 1 bedroom apartment available so I signed the lease and got on an airplane to start my new life.

Moving to a whole new city without knowing anyone was exciting but despite making some really great friends, I was missing the feeling of closeness that I got from being around my family. On the fourth of July I went for a walk around the trail near my apartment and I remember seeing all of these couples that looked so happy and it broke my heart because I had never experienced that and wanted it so bad. I went home and prayed for a girlfriend that night. A few days later I was doing a live-stream and got a comment from the most beautiful girl I had ever seen that said "How many carbs are in do you have a girlfriend?". This was probably the most exciting moment of my life because it felt like my prayer was being answered.

After the live ended I messaged the girl who sent it and explained to her that I really didn't want to use my platform for dating but this felt like it was meant to happen. Ana and I immediately started talking on FaceTime every day because she lived in New York and I lived in Texas but after a few months she came to visit me for an entire month in September of 2020. She liked Austin so much that she found an apartment the third week she was here and signed a lease to move in by november.

While being in a relationship brought me a level of happiness that I had never experienced, it also came with its challenges. For example: I realized that I had an anxious attachment style. Which basically means that when she had to return to New York after her visit and prepare for the move here, I spent an entire month worrying that she might never come back. I had no reason to believe that was the case but this type of anxiety is really good at over-powering the rational part of your brain that knows everything is going to be fine. Despite all of this anxiety I was dealing with, I never once had the thought of using food to make myself feel better which would have been my go-to a few years ago. I instead developed coping mechanisms like going for long walks and catching up with friends.

Coping mechanisms are something that can either be really beneficial or really unhealthy and most of us develop the unhealthy ones without even realizing it. As I reflect on the experience of healing my relationship with food in the beginning of my keto journey, I can see that I was undoing an unhealthy coping mechanism I developed in child-hood and replacing it with things like meditation, exercise and being part of a community. So if food is always the solution to negative emotions, you might want to look for other ways of dealing with those emotions. Therapy is a great resource for this.

Another challenge that came with being in a relationship was the fact that instead of spending all of my time making keto recipes and creating content I actually had to do things like go out to dinner and travel. These things are normal to the average person but I was so focused on my mission that it was kind of a culture shock to step outside of the Keto Instagram world. However, I was able to maintain my abstinence from carbs for the most part.

Chapter 10: Relapse

Finally in June of 2021 I ended my streak of 2 years without a cheat day. I had experienced a few higher carb meals during the period leading up to this but I never went off for an entire day. I honestly just didn't have the desire to. However this time was different. We were traveling to New York for Ana's brother's graduation and I gave myself a 3 day pass to shove all of the junk into my mouth.

The first meal did have rice, but it wasn't junk food at all because it was home cooked Peruvian food that Ana's mom made. Which was incredible! But the next day the carb fest began. We went to explore New York City and I started out by eating a hot dog and a piece of pizza. They were amazing. Then we went to the Museum of Ice Cream and that was even better. Finally we went to an Italian restaurant and I was in heaven. By the end of the trip I had stuffed myself to the max and was ready to get back on Keto.

Then over the next few months we took 2 more trips where my 3 day free passes started to become a problem. My weight was slowly creeping up from 170 to 180 and my loyalty to keto was starting to slip. I didn't have a problem staying keto most of the time, but after experiencing all of my favorite comfort foods again I wanted to have more cheats. Which sent my satisfaction with keto food way down.

This is a major problem that a lot of people on their weight loss journey will run into. The more often you eat highly palatable junk food, the less you appreciate the healthy foods that you are supposed to be eating. During the 2 years of my carb abstinence you couldn't have told me that a low carb tortilla pizza wasn't as good as a piece of pizza from pizza hut. Or that a pint of rebel ice cream wasn't better than a blizzard. But after experiencing these foods so frequently again, I remembered what it was like to fight carb cravings.

In December 2021 I realized it was time to take things with Ana to the next level so I went ring shopping, found the perfect one and bought it. My plan was to hold onto it until February and propose to her during our trip to Cabo for my birthday. But I was so excited after picking up the ring that holding it in was causing me to lose my mind. Everytime I thought about proposing I would start crying and then she would ask why I was crying, which meant I had to start making up reasons. I was a wreck. So 3 days later on December 19th we were getting ready to go out and I couldn't wait any longer. I got on one knee in the kitchen and proposed. She said yes and I was filled with joy but also kicking myself for not making it at least a little more special. But she wanted it to be a surprise and with her constant probing about why I was always crying, I didn't have much time left.

3 weeks later I woke up on an ordinary Sunday, met with a friend for some coffee and came home to a very different Ana than I was used to. I'm not sure what it was but something about her was giving me a weird vibe. Not in a bad way, if anything it was a good vibe. I even remember she looked extra beautiful. There was a special glow about her. So after coming in and getting settled she told me that Harley, our dog, had something for me. So I walked over to her and underneath the dog was a pregnancy test. It was positive. I was overwhelmed with joy. Rather than being scared or nervous, it was like everything in my life clicked and my purpose felt more clear than ever. It suddenly felt like my life wasn't about me anymore, and it was almost a relief. I can't explain it to this day but it feels like the day I truly "grew up".

The next 9 months were a wild ride. Ana actually did keto for the first month, but once those pregnancy cravings hit it was a wrap. So now my increased desire for cheat days was being tested by many more opportunities to eat off plan than I was used to. Whether it was the trips to Walgreens for her favorite treats or the dinners out where she ordered sweet potato fries AND dessert, I was struggling. It never got to the point where I cheated more than once a week but it felt like my relationship with food was regressing to where it was at the beginning of my keto journey.

Another thing that happened during pregnancy was finding out that the baby was measuring small at our anatomy scan. To make things even more dramatic, the doctor who broke the news to us had a very cold russian accent. He started explaining all of the risks and told us that if she stops growing at any point in the pregnancy we will have to deliver immediately. We were shook to the core. It turns out that many people have this experience because if a doctor notices one small abnormality they have to give you a plethora of scary information to avoid being sued. The last thing he told us was that we have to come in for weekly ultrasounds for the rest of the pregnancy to make sure the baby is healthy.

Things did get better though because the next week we saw a super upbeat doctor who assured us that things like this happen all the time and the vast majority of people in our situation deliver a healthy baby. And the week after that we spoke with a neonatologist who gave us even more positive reassurance by telling us that he was in the exact same place as us with one of his children and everything turned out fine. There was something about his story that really hit me in the heart and made me feel like everything was going to be okay. Even though the first doctor with the off-putting tone of voice also told us we would more than likely deliver a healthy baby, it was the personal story and positive energy that eased my anxiety.

So every week that we went to the doctor we tried our best to stay positive but it was challenging. Especially in the beginning when an early delivery was a lot more risky. If I thought that finding out we were having a baby caused me to grow up, this added another 20 years to my emotional growth spurt. But every week that she looked healthy, was another week that our baby got to stay safe and sound in the womb! By 34 weeks she was still growing and we had reached the golden zone where an early delivery is extremely safe.

Despite all of this emotional turbulence, I am proud to say that none of the cheating I did during pregnancy was out of emotional distress. So while it felt like the weekly cheats were 2016 all over again, they actually weren't because this time around I had much more control over when they happened, and how much I allowed myself to have.

Here is what a cheat day looked like during pregnancy:

I would start my day by putting a protein shake in my coffee, then have some eggs and bacon for lunch which was my usual routine regardless of whether I was cheating or not. Finally dinner would be my biggest meal and depending on the restaurant we went to I might order a steak with fries and mac n cheese. However, I am notorious for having a second dinner before bed so after we got home I would often walk to the Dairy Queen next to our house and get a chicken basket with a small blizzard.

Compared to the cheat days I was having in 2016, you can see that I really did have a much healthier strategy for going off plan. The key to preventing an all out binge was likely the fact that I kept the first half of my day high in protein and consistent with my usual eating habits. It's important for anyone, on any eating plan to always start the day with something high in protein. Because protein sets a hormonal cascade into motion that will make it significantly easier to avoid over-eating throughout the rest of the day.

Then on August 25th Sofia Aleni Wiggins was born and that was truly the greatest day of my life. I thought that finding out Ana was pregnant changed me as a man, but finally holding Sofia and feeling her grasp onto my finger with her tiny little hand was a totally different experience. It was like my entire sense of self disappeared and the only thing left was love. Realizing that the well-being of this little human was 100% our responsibility felt like the greatest gift in the world.

Eventually the magic wore off and we returned home along with my sense of self. But I will forever be transformed by that experience. Every moment I spend with Sofia still feels like a gift and it is just such a blessing to take care of her, even when she is driving us insane.

Chapter 11: Baby Weight Be Gone

The hospital stay was such a beautiful experience that despite eating off plan for pretty much every meal, I never ordered seconds or thirds. I was so amazed by this love bubble that the three of us were existing in that it didn't feel it was necessary to eat a ton of food. However, after returning home I spent another week eating off plan for basically every meal. That's when I realized I had ballooned up to 195 lbs, which is the most I've weighed since losing weight the first time around.

Ana & I were both ready to get back on track so we stayed on plan for almost 2 months but my weight wasn't moving much. That's when I made it a priority to lift more weights, walk more often and cut back on the fun keto foods like low carb bread and tortillas. This helped a bit but it just felt like my body wanted to stay at 190. I actually don't have a problem with my body at 190 lbs but after doing keto for so many years it felt like my body was challenging me to push a little harder. Coincidentally I had just listened to a podcast that totally changed my perspective on calorie counting. So I decided that on top of doing keto I would also track my calories for a week as an experiment.

WARNING: I transformed my eating habits and got to a healthy weight by focusing on carbs and carbs alone. So please do not read this and assume that I am pushing calorie counting as something beginners have to do. It can be very stressful, especially for sedentary women who have much lower caloric needs than someone like me. If you are 300 lbs and want to be at a healthy weight, focusing on carbs will likely get you there. Calorie counting from my experience is often only necessary to drop the last 10-15 lbs.

Going into this I made it very clear that I would never let an app tell me I wasn't allowed to eat if I was hungry. Whether I was 200 or 2,000 calories over it didn't matter. I was going to eat if I felt like I needed to. So I downloaded MyFitnessPal, which sucks for tracking net carbs by the way, but is otherwise easy to use. Based on my information the app told me I could eat 2,600 calories per day if I wanted to lose ½ lb per week. I wasn't sure what 2,600 calories looked like so I didn't know whether to be scared or excited.

I quickly realized that 2,600 calories can either be a ton of food or very little food depending on what you eat. For example, a huge plate of chicken breast with sugar free ketchup and steamed carrots has less calories than a candy bar. This is when I started looking into volume eating, which got me pretty excited about my calorie counting experiment. Volume eating is basically where you eat low calorie, high volume foods such as lean protein, high fiber veggies & berries. However, going all in on volume eating would have conflicted with my belief that a high fat intake is also important for living a low carb lifestyle.

So I sort of blended the two together in a way that allows for maximum satiation while not dropping my fat intake too low. A day of eating basically looked like: Coffee with a protein shake for breakfast. Something a bit higher in fat for lunch such as an omelette with peppers, onions & spinach cooked in butter. And for dinner I would go pretty high on volume with a big plate of chicken breast dipped in sugar free ketchup. Air fried broccoli, lightly coated with avocado oil. 2-3 servings of mashed cauliflower without adding too much butter or heavy cream. Low carb yogurt with a scoop of protein powder and a lot of mixed berries. And for snacks throughout the day I was turning to grape tomatoes rather than cheese cubes or pork rinds.

This way of eating did make it a bit harder to achieve deep ketosis, but I was still measuring around 0.7 on my keto meter so I wasn't worried about it too much. I was also feeling much more full at the end of the day than I did with my usual approach to keto so rather than ending my day at 2,600 calories, it was often around 2,200. After 3 weeks of tracking something crazy happened. I decided to weigh myself and was down to 183.

This made it extremely hard to not run and tell my audience that keto alone isn't enough, you also have to track your calories! But I knew better than that because I remember how I felt as a beginner when people told me to track my calories. It felt like they were telling me to go run a marathon with no training. But based on this little experiment, my view on weight loss will never be the same. Like I mentioned, I still believe that counting carbs is enough to make massive changes to your health and your body composition. But I now understand that calorie counting is an incredible tool that gives you complete control over how much weight you can lose. Especially when paired with keto.

As I am writing this, most of the baby weight is gone and I don't feel the need to continue tracking calories. I simply don't find it to be a necessary means of maintaining a healthy weight if I'm already doing keto, assuming we don't get pregnant and go carb crazy again! Plus, the main thing that I took away from it is similar to what I learned from carb counting at the beginning of my keto journey. Which is basically knowing when to indulge and when to be mindful of serving sizes. Because low volume, high calorie foods like ranch dressing can add up very quickly.

As far as the rest of my life, things are great all around. Sofia is healthy and sleeping 12 hours through the night which feels like a miracle. My career as a keto personality is taking me places I never imagined possible. And I am so excited to bring you guys along for the rest of my journey as KetoSnackz!

What now?

Now that you know all about keto, my story & what it means to live a "Care Free Keto" lifestyle, let's get into the rest of the book! I will start out by explaining how you can take baby steps towards getting healthy and then we will get into the food!

PART 3 YOUR TRANSFORMATION

This is the part of the book where we talk about baby-stepping your way into a healthy lifestyle and I guide you on your transformation!

Chapter 12: Baby Steps

Three steps to go from carb-addict to success story

Most people hear keto success stories and are drawn to them because they want to succeed too, but they don't know where to start so they never do. Or they do start but set themselves up for failure by getting information from all over the internet and believe they can only eat beef, butter, & mayonnaise. It feels very overwhelming to go from eating anything you want to all of a sudden having to count every carb you eat. The truth is that you don't have to quit carbs cold turkey.

While it is necessary to limit your carbs to around 25g per day to get into ketosis, you don't have to start your health journey with ketosis as the goal. Instead of starting with something you know you won't stick to, utilize the power of baby steps and start with something attainable. This will allow you to create healthy habits that will slowly but surely turn you into the type of person who CAN stick to 25g of net carbs per day.

Before getting started, it's important to know that you might not see much weight-loss until you get to the second and third baby steps. However, the first step is often an essential step that will help you establish a healthy relationship with food. For example; When I was getting started, had I not been adding blueberries to my milkshakes or adding avocado to my breakfasts, I wouldn't have undergone the identity shift that was so essential in finally cutting out unhealthy foods. This is a game of believing in yourself, because the story you tell yourself about why you can or can't do something can either be the most limiting or empowering thing in your life.

Another thing to consider is that baby steps might not be for you! If you have experience counting carbs and eating healthy, there is nothing wrong with jumping into 25g net carbs per day, counting every calorie and working out like an athlete! Extreme approaches like this may not work for the average person but if you want to change badly enough, I truly believe you can start and stick to anything!

> Feel free to start with baby step #1 for a few weeks and then take the other steps at your own pace, or jump ahead as far as you want! This is not a one size fits all approach.

Baby step #1 - Adding:

Unlearn the restrictive nature of diets & focus on adding foods to your diet that make you feel healthy

How to "add" - Pick a food or food group that makes you feel healthy, and consume it every day! It's that easy

The main excuse that holds us back is the belief that we are not capable of change. And the more often we try & fail miserably, the stronger that excuse becomes. So in order to weaken it we need to find proof that it is not true. But the harsh reality is that most of us are not yet capable of giving up the foods that bring us joy. Otherwise we would have given them up a long time ago. So knowing that we probably won't succeed if we just jump straight into restricting, the question is... what can we do? This is where "adding" comes in to save the day!

Simply add one healthy thing to one of your meals each day, with an emphasis on things that make YOU feel healthy. While I currently believe that aiming for 30g+ of protein at each meal is the optimal approach to adding, maybe you feel healthy by adding berries to your oatmeal in the morning. That is totally fine. The point is for you to start feeling like someone who is capable of making changes towards improving their health. This will break down the excuse that you aren't the type of person who can get healthy, and that is a HUGE STEP!

After you succeed with adding one healthy item to one meal each day, I encourage you to continue the process of adding healthy things to all of your meals while you're taking the next steps! Or if this one really jives with you, maybe you won't feel the need to take the next steps because there is simply no room for unhealthy foods on your plate!

The last piece of advice that will make this step more effective is to eat the healthy foods that you decide to add FIRST! For example.. If you add half an avocado to your breakfast, eat the avocado first. That way the blood sugar spike from the carbs you eat will be much less severe, minimizing the crash later on that causes cravings. This works because fiber slows down the rate at which your body processes the rest of your food. So when you are eating a meal higher in carbs, starting out with fiber is essential for stable blood sugar. It can also help fill you up before deciding to finish the rest of the unhealthy foods in that meal!

Here is an example of what ADDING can look like based on someone who eats a diet pretty high in junk food.

Week one - Adding to one meal each day

Breakfast	Pancakes, bacon & half an avocado.	Adds - Half an avocado for the fiber and healthy fats at the beginning of the meal, reducing the amount of pancakes they need to feel satisfied.

Week two - Adding to two meals each day

Breakfast	Bowl of fruity pebbles and 2 hard boiled eggs.	Adds - The hard boiled eggs for the protein and fats that will curb the desire for a second bowl of cereal.
Lunch	Pasta, breadsticks and grilled chicken salad.	Adds - Grilled chicken salad for the protein and fiber that prevents the overconsumption of breadsticks.

Week three - Adding to three meals each day

Breakfast	Eggs, biscuits with grape jam & bowl of berries.	Adds - Adds berries for the fiber and as a way to satisfy their sweet tooth, curbing the overconsumption of biscuits
Lunch	Cheeseburger, fries and side salad.	Adds - Side salad for the fiber that helps fill them up and reduce the amount of fries needed to feel satisfied.
Dinner	Pork chops with green beans and mashed potatoes.	Adds - Extra serving of green beans to help curb the desire for a big dessert later on.

By week four they are adding healthy foods to each meal and even adding plain greek yogurt with berries to their dessert routine, which results in eating less cookies. Their overall caloric intake is starting to decrease because the fiber, protein and healthy fats they are eating at each meal is making it easier to resist mindless snacking throughout the day.

Katie's story:

A perfect example of how powerful "adding" can be is the story of my friend, Katie.

Katie struggled with her weight her entire life & everytime she tried to make a change she could never stick to it. After years of feeling defeated she read a book called "Atomic Habits" that showed her the power of making changes by starting with small habits. This book inspired her to start her health journey with something she KNEW she could stick to. So instead of attempting to eat 1200 calories a day all week only to binge all weekend, she simply decided to start each day with a green smoothie. (Personally, I don't think that green smoothies are the move.. But if that makes you feel healthy then more power to you)

After weeks of drinking these green smoothies, Katie's feelings about herself started to change. Instead of the helpless feeling she was used to, she started to feel like the type of person who can set a goal and actually stick to it. Even though she was still eating Chick-Fil-A for lunch & frozen pizza for dinner, she had finally created this one positive habit that made her believe she is in fact capable of change!

The next baby step she took was replacing her favorite snack, potato chips, with beef sticks and nuts. After that she replaced her favorite carb filled side dishes at dinner with vegetables. Fast forward two years and she was 100 pounds lighter happily living a low carb lifestyle! The journey definitely wasn't a smooth ride to perfect health as she would occasionally back track, but she started with the smallest step possible and totally transformed herself into the person she always wanted to be.

Baby step #2 - Weaning:

We know that sugar is as addictive as drugs, yet we expect people to quit cold turkey... That is crazy!

How to "wean" - Slowly wean yourself off of carbs by eliminating the obvious carbs from one meal each day!

The next excuse that holds us back is the belief that we love eating junk! While it is true that we get pleasure from junk food, unless we enjoy being diagnosed with pre-diabetes, not fitting into the jeans we want to wear & the rest of the baggage that comes from being overweight we can't honestly say that we "love" the food that got us there! The worst part is.. Even after coming to this realization and committing to a healthy lifestyle, our brain is going to fight and fight to hold on to that little bit of joy we get from the junk food we're used to eating. After all, SUGAR IS ADDICTING! So instead of quitting cold Turkey this step will show you how to start slow and wean yourself off of the carbs, with the option to still eat the late night brownie if you're craving it.

Start by selecting one meal per day & making it as low carb as possible. You don't even have to count the carbs, just get rid of the bread, pasta, rice, etc.. It also helps to make sure that this is a protein packed meal so you don't end up with more cravings 3 hours later. For example; If you are used to starting the day with a bowl of lucky charms or a pastry, which is literally dessert by the way. Try starting the day with eggs, bacon & half an avocado. And if that doesn't satisfy your sweet tooth, have some berries at the end. This breakfast will boost your mood, minimize cravings throughout the day & it will taste awesome!

After a few weeks of this, the "win" of knowing that you are capable of sticking to one low carb meal per day will totally change the way you view yourself. This is the most rewarding part & it's important to celebrate it. Even if you are still eating junk after dinner, you did make a change when you thought it was impossible to change! That is huge. This change in the way you view yourself will give you the confidence and momentum to try going for 2 healthy meals each day! And eventually you can start cutting out the obvious carbs from every meal you eat.

The best part is that as you remove more and more unhealthy meals from your day and replace them with healthy meals, you will typically start dreading the bowl of spaghetti for dinner because you know how crappy it's going to make you feel. And once you start associating junk food with feeling crappy, it gets easier and easier to take control of your eating habits!

The last tip for this baby step is to start with breakfast and incorporate protein if you can. When you start your day with a high protein, low carb meal you are setting yourself up for stable blood sugar throughout the day. This along with the many other hormonal benefits of getting adequate protein will make it significantly easier to make healthy choices around food the rest of the day.

Here is an example of someone who is following the weaning plan:

Week one - Removes from one meal each day

Breakfast	Eggs, bacon & half an avocado.	Removes - Toast, resulting in more stable blood sugar and less cravings the rest of the day.

Week two - Removes from two meals each day

Breakfast	Bowl of unflavored yogurt with berries & protein powder.	Removes - French toast sticks, which usually lead to a plate of seconds that wasn't due to hunger but simply because they tasted so good.
Lunch	Grilled nuggets & side salad.	Removes - Fries, which prevents the post meal crash that usually requires a sugary coffee to bring their energy levels back up.

Week three - Removes from three meals each day

Breakfast	Cheese stick, beef jerky & mixed veggies.	Removes - Flavored crackers that usually caused the overconsumption of everything else due to palatability.
Lunch	Large salmon salad with olive oil dressing.	Removes - Soda that almost always resulted in a refill on the way out of the restaurant.
Dinner	Steak with roasted carrots and cauliflower mash.	Removes - Dinner rolls that would result in craving something sweet later on and eating too many oreos.

Baby step #3 - Counting:

Counting carbs is the most important step for getting & staying in ketosis. This is where you can expect the weight-loss to really speed up as well!

Before reading this section, I feel that it's important for me to keep reminding you that being in ketosis is not the only way to lose weight and improve your health. If you simply learn to count your carbs & stay under 30, 50, or even 100, you may achieve the goals you desire and feel no need to get into ketosis. The same applies to calories. That is totally fine!

How to "count" -

You already learned to count net carbs in the first chapter of the book, so here is a reminder of the formula:

total carbs - fiber - sugar alcohols - allulose = net carbs

Whether you're using an app or the notepad on your iPhone, you simply want to keep track of the net carbs from each meal and make sure to stay under 25g net carbs for the day. See an example below!

Breakfast -
3 eggs with salsa: 2g net carbs
Half an avocado: 2g net carbs

Lunch -
Caesar salad: 5g net carbs
Serving of walnuts: 2g net carbs

Dinner -
Chicken thighs: 0g net carbs
Brussels sprouts: 8g net carbs

Dessert -
Raspberries: 4g net carbs

After a few days of tracking, you may find that you're eating WAY more carbs than you assumed, or maybe you're eating an average of 20g per day which is great! The typical beginner will want to stay under 25g net carbs per day in order to reach a state of ketosis. However, if you start logging your carbs and realize you're consuming 100+ carbs per day despite cutting out bread, pasta, & rice from the majority of your meals. There is no shame in baby stepping your way down to 25g net carbs per day from 100! Simply reduce the number by 20 each week, and eventually you will be doing 25g per day without too much of a struggle.

Once you're down to 25g net carbs per day, you can start testing your ketones. This is NOT required for success, but it is helpful! The basic rules for testing ketones are as follows:

1. Use a blood ketone monitor, not urine strips.

2. Give yourself 2 hours after eating, working out or waking up before testing.

3. Test daily for the first week, every other day for the second week, and eventually you can just do weekly tests to be sure you haven't added anything into your diet that's interfering with ketosis.

The first few weeks that you're in ketosis the weight will typically be coming off FAST. Don't get too excited because it's mostly water weight. After the rapid weight loss phase is over, the average person can expect to lose ½ pound to 2 pounds per week depending on how much they have to lose.

Now you did it! You baby stepped your way into Ketosis! Congratulations.

Chapter 13: Love Yourself First

Now that you've read my story, the basics of keto and how to ease into this lifestyle, you might be wondering... "How much weight am I going to lose? How long will it take? I'm ready for MY keto transformation!"

We will get to that in the next chapter. But before we talk about tracking progress and how much weight-loss you can expect to see, it's very important for you to look in the mirror and commit to taking care of yourself as the first priority. While being overweight is not the healthiest state for your body to be in, being consumed by self-hate isn't either. So if you simply can't find the strength to love yourself, let's talk about how you got to where you are and why it truly isn't your fault...

As we discussed previously, the junk food that fills your pantry and refrigerator was designed to be overconsumed & most of us have been encouraged to eat it our entire lives. There is a great book called "The Dorito Effect" that explains how most food companies use artificial flavors to make their products more appealing, and this flavoring of processed food decreases our desire to eat real, whole food. And anyone who has dabbled in calorie counting will have a clear understanding of why this would cause wide-spread weight gain.

For example; Imagine one person drinks a sugary coffee for breakfast with a bacon egg and cheese biscuit. Then for lunch they get a Big Mac meal with a medium fry and a medium soda. Dinner is a frozen pizza and maybe they want something sweet before bed so they eat a bowl of cereal. Now imagine another person starts their day with scrambled eggs, bacon, sliced bell peppers and coffee with a little milk. For lunch they have a pork chop with a loaded baked potato and dinner is a large salmon salad with balsamic vinaigrette. Maybe they also want something sweet before bed so let's say they had greek yogurt with a cup of berries.

Despite the fact that they both seem to be eating 3 filling meals, the first person is easily consuming an extra 300 calories per day. And if a surplus of 3,500 calories = 1 pound of fat storage, the first person will gain an extra 30 lbs in just 1 year.

So for those of us who grew up eating fast food and think of processed food as "normal food" we are literally destined for weight gain. And it's not easy to just label processed food as bad and stop eating it. So what do we do? While the weight-gain may not be our fault entirely, that doesn't mean it's not our job to fix it. Unless we can wait long enough for a new obesity drug to come and save us. The key is to recognize that your taste buds have been compromised and apply the baby steps mentality to changing them back to their natural state.

The second thing working against us is that we are stuck with the same brain that humans evolved to have 100,000 years ago, when high calorie foods were scarce. It wasn't until very recently that we gained access to an abundance of food & our brains simply haven't had time to adjust. Maybe 100,000 years from now the ability to stop eating when satiated will become a built in mechanism used to push the species forward.. But for now we have the same instincts that allowed us to thrive in a food-scarce environment, an environment where not having the urge to binge on high calorie foods would be a disadvantage.

So next time you find yourself overeating or cheating on your diet, please remember that it is not a personality flaw. It is actually a strength that allowed our ancestors to survive. It's just not very useful anymore. So acknowledging this is a great way to combat the self-hate a lot of us feel for being overweight. The best way to override these instincts is to fill up on nutrient dense foods and limit your exposure to your trigger foods.

Chapter 14: Progress

Now that you finally love yourself, or at least understand how a big part of weight gain is not due to some flaw within us. Let's talk about tracking progress and how much of it to expect.

Below are my 2 favorite approaches to tracking progress.

Approach 1: Tracking your inches

So once you've taken all the baby steps the best approach to tracking progress is simply measuring your inches once a month. You can use measuring tape or a fun way to visualize your results is to use a piece of yarn and hang it on the wall each month. The reason I find this to be the best approach is because the scale can be deceiving. Things like bloating, not using the bathroom and random fluctuations can convince you that you are not losing weight even if you actually are. That can really become a problem if you're an emotional eater.

For example; A follower of mine messaged me in 2020 after going off the rails for 8 months. She gained back the 30 lbs she lost in her first year of keto plus an extra 10. She told me that this whole chain of events started because she weighed in on a Friday and saw that she was up 3 lbs from her Monday weigh in. That led to stress eating junk food all weekend, making the not so wise decision of weighing in again on Sunday and ultimately giving up.

If you have ever had an experience like this, or if you are particularly sensitive to the scale I highly recommend going the route of tracking your inches.

Approach 2: Weekly average

The next best approach is to confront the weight fluctuations head on and weigh yourself every day... But what you are going to do is take the average weight for each week and log that as your progress. This way you will become aware of how often the scale fluctuates and seeing that you're up 3 lbs on a random Tuesday won't send you into a downward spiral!

Here is an example:

Day 1: 182.6

Day 2: 184.1

Day 3: 182.4

Day 4: 181.6

Day 5: 183.2

Day 6: 181.8

Day 7: 181

Total: 182.6 + 184.1 + 182.4 + 181.6 + 183.2 + 181.8 + 181 = 1,276.9

Average: 1,276.9 / 7 = 182.4

So with this formula your average weight for the week is 182.4 This number minimizes the emotional turbulence that is often experienced during weigh-ins because you are focused on the weekly average, not the fluctuations that can be very scary at times!

After you pick a plan for tracking progress, it's time to manage your expectations of progress.. Because the truth is that everyone's weight loss will happen at a different pace and the more anxious you are about seeing massive results, the more unstable you are going to feel throughout this journey. You want to be as calm and in control as possible so that when the cravings come you can resist them. And stepping on the scale every day expecting to see results, is going to make you feel anything but calm and in control.

MY WEIGHT-LOSS

First let's talk about MY weight-loss. Below are the 3 main reasons how keto helped ME lose 80 lbs in 2 years.

1. Lowering my carb intake reduced my options to primarily meat and veggies. These foods weren't as fun to overeat as grilled cheese sandwiches and candy bars but were still enjoyable enough for me to eat long-term.

2. Protein, fat and fiber from real foods are much more satiating than processed grains and sugar. And the more satiated I felt, the less likely I was to overeat.

3. Keto kept my blood sugar stable, which helped me avoid the burning desire to eat the entire pantry that came after a blood sugar crash. Stable blood sugar was also great for my mental health, which made it easier to control my food choices.

As you can see, all three of these examples come back to one thing: LESS OVEREATING

While many Instagram gurus will tell you that not eating enough fat is the cause of your weight gain, the truth is that overeating is the driver of weight gain. It's just that a diet high in fat and protein is great at curbing the excessive hunger that leads to overeating. And while using keto to reduce insulin and bringing balance to other obesity driving hormones can be helpful, it will never give you the same results as simply not overeating. So rather than viewing keto as a magic pill that causes rapid weight loss, it's helpful to view it as a tool that reduces your appetite and creates the ideal conditions for weight-loss. But simply being in ketosis will not always get you to your goal, even if it gets you pretty close.

YOUR WEIGHT-LOSS

Assuming that you stick to keto the majority of the time and are eating the right foods you probably will see a lot of weight loss during the first month. It's very motivating to see the scale dropping 3, 4 or even 5 lbs per week. The problem is, the weight loss during the first month is not primarily fat. Your body gets rid of a lot of stored water when you stop eating carbs and that can be up to 20 lbs for some! After this you can expect to lose anything between 0.5 and 3 lbs per week. If you have a lot of weight to lose, you may experience more but that is in the case of people who are 100+ lbs overweight.

The average person looking to lose 30-40 lbs will probably lose around 1 lb per week. Which is pretty hard to accept after the huge drop in water weight the first few weeks.

One thing that can help you stay positive during this phase of weight loss is to remember that most people who take extreme measures to lose a ton of weight very quickly, are often the same people who gain it back even faster. The more sustainable your approach is and the lower your expectations are, the more likely you are to actually stay on track and eventually get to your goal.

However, if you spend several months without the scale moving, my best advice is to first start tracking your inches. Because many people, especially those without much weight to lose in the first place will actually find that their body is shrinking despite the fact that the scale isn't moving. This is because when you follow a keto diet your body increases growth hormone, which increases lean body mass even if you aren't lifting weights. So someone with 15 lbs to lose who is mildly active might actually put on some muscle, burn some fat and wear a smaller jean size despite the scale not reflecting it. If this is the case, I recommend using inches rather than weight to track progress.

If the inches aren't going down either, it's likely due to overeating or falling off track too often. The next 2 chapters are a great resource for overcoming a plateau.

Chapter 15: Lifestyle Habits & Food Cravings

What if you took all of the baby steps & you're eating the right food, but it still feels like a struggle to stay on track? Or maybe you are staying on track but the weight just isn't coming off.. That's where this chapter helps!

It's important to know that certain lifestyle habits can make your journey feel 100 times easier & other lifestyle habits can make it feel impossible to turn down junk food. I wholeheartedly believe that we aren't born with a set amount of will-power & destined to be successful or unsuccessful. It's much more likely that we are born with varying levels of will-power that can fluctuate based on lifestyle habits. Below are some of the most important habits that can influence the types of food you crave and how much food you end up eating.

Habit #1 - SLEEP

Studies show that poor sleep quality ramps up the hormones that make you feel hungry & down regulates the hormones that make you feel satiated after a meal.

Studies also show that eating large meals & viewing bright lights (TV, phone screen, bright bathroom lights) before bedtime can impair your sleep quality. All of which are more common than not in our current society. Which begs the question, is the REAL

YOU always hungry or is the version of you with altered hormones always hungry?

Here are my tips on improving your sleep habits.

1. **Get outside as soon as you wake up** - Because the first 10 minutes that are spent outside each day will set your circadian clock, signaling to your brain that it's time to get tired in 12 hours. This is especially helpful if you have trouble falling asleep. It even works on cloudy days!

2. **Dim the lights after 9 PM** - When you see bright lights before bed it disrupts the sleepy chemicals in your brain, which also disrupts your happy chemicals. I personally recommend wearing blue light blocking glasses, but be sure to get the amber tinted ones for maximum effectiveness!

3. **Supplement Magnesium** - Magnesium is responsible for many things in the body and one of them is feeling relaxed. If you're deficient, every night will feel like a battle trying to fall asleep. This is the most important thing I've ever done for my sleep. I take 400 mg magnesium glycinate every night.

4. **Hydrate early** - If you wait until 10 PM to properly hydrate yourself, you will be peeing all night. I try to cut back on fluids 1-2 hours before bed & right before going to sleep I take 1-2 tsp of salt, this has made a big difference in how often I wake up to pee!

5. **Stop using food as a sleep ai**d - Going to sleep right after eating isn't the end of the world, but unfortunately it does lower sleep quality. And if you're like me who grew up eating a bowl of cereal or cookies right before bed, you probably feel like you can't get sleepy without eating something. My strategy is simply to make sure I eat a pretty big meal 3-4 hours before bed & allow snacks 1-2 hours before bed. That way when the cravings come I don't feel hungry enough to give in!

Habit #2 - Emotional management

Emotional eating is REAL and if the only tool you have to feel better after a bad day is taking a trip to McDonald's, you're not alone. However, there are better ways to cope with negative emotions.

Disclaimer: If you have serious mental health concerns, seek professional help. This is simply a list of emotional management strategies that I wish someone gave me when I was first starting out on my keto journey.

1. **Journaling** - Simply spend 2, 10, or 30 minutes writing whatever is on your mind. This is helpful because whatever is bothering us, is usually a much bigger problem in our head than it is in reality. When we realize this truth, our feelings have much less power over us and are less likely to drive us into making poor food choices. Journaling is also a helpful tool to remind yourself of your goals and why they are important to you. If you decide to write down your "why" every time you feel tempted and then journal about all of the reasons reaching that goal is important to you, amazing things can start happening for you!

2. **Meditation** - Sit down and focus on your breath or repeat a mantra for any amount of time that you feel comfortable with. The goal is 20 minutes but when you're first starting out, even 3 minutes is an accomplishment. Meditation has been shown in countless studies to make us less impulsive, less anxious, and less stressed which makes it A LOT easier to turn down junk food when we feel tempted!

3. **Long walks** - The same way that meditation reduces stress & anxiety, so does going for walks! You can actually turn off the part of your brain that sends you into fight or flight mode during stressful situations by going for a walk outside.

4. **Exercise** - Whatever emotional issues you're dealing with can probably be resolved with exercise. It doesn't matter what you do, just move your body! Our brains evolved as part of a physically active body and when we neglect physical activity, the brain isn't able to do its job in keeping us happy and emotionally healthy.

5. **Connection** - It's amazing how great we feel after spending quality time with (the right) people. Just be sure to avoid planning this quality time around the consumption of crappy food. If that means meeting up at a park instead of going for tacos and margaritas, your friends will understand!

Habit #3 - Food selection

The food you eat (or don't eat) can make it easier or harder to stay on track. Things like sugary processed foods that are designed to be overconsumed can spike your blood sugar which sets you up for cravings all day, while other foods high in protein can satiate you throughout the day.

1. **Start your day with protein & fat** - Whether you're two weeks into keto or on your first baby step towards living healthier, filling up with protein and fat will 100% make it easier to turn down junk food the rest of the day.

2. **Avoid the "just a bite" lie we tell ourselves** - This is especially true if you're cooking & buying snacks for your family. One bite of Mac N' Cheese is rarely one bite. And when you've had 4 massive bites of Mac N' Cheese you can almost certainly expect cravings for the rest of the day. You don't need to torture yourself like that.

3. **Get out of your comfort zone in the kitchen** - When you get a craving for pizza, it's possible to just push it down and try to distract yourself from it. But sometimes these cravings are too hard to resist and we give in.. Instead of fighting the craving, just make a keto version! It won't be as delicious & it might be a bit challenging to make, but it is definitely an easier option than relying on will-power & self restraint.

4. **Don't be afraid of keto snacks** - Similar to the above tip, this will help you deal with cravings in a sustainable way. I personally eat an enlightened ice cream bar every night to satisfy my sweet tooth. There may be a time and a place to cut out keto snacks in order to speed up weight loss, but if you're barely hanging on at the beginning of your health journey this is probably not the time!

5. **Do or don't try Intermittent fasting** - In the keto space a lot of people assume they have to do intermittent fasting too, which can make this already difficult lifestyle change way too overwhelming. While it is an effective tool for some people to control their appetite, others just end up binge eating junk food at the end of the day. Listen to your body and realize that you DO NOT have to do intermittent fasting, but you can if it feels right for you!

Habit #4 - Finding your people

One of the greatest truths I've ever heard is this... You become the 5 people you spend the most time with. The hardest but most effective way to upgrade your habits is to upgrade your friend group, so if you can go out into the world and make friends with people who are a little further ahead than you it will be a game changer. However, the way I started was simply by finding the right podcasts to listen to, content creators to watch and authors to read. There are an abundance of positive influences to surround yourself with on the internet!

1. **Podcasts / Books** - If you don't have a lot of positive influences in your life, the best place to start is through books & podcasts. When I first started listening to podcasts my entire philosophy on life shifted. Podcasts sparked my interest in audiobooks and that's how I gained the tools to really change my life.

2. **Social Media** - If you go on social media and it is filled with doom and gloom, here is what I want you to do. Everytime you see a post that makes you feel bad, unfollow that account. Even if you value knowing what's going on in the world, social media is not the place to learn about it. Replace these accounts with educational / inspirational people who are promoting the lifestyle you aspire to live. Be careful not to compare yourself to these people though because we are all on our own journey and your day 9 looks a lot different than someone else's day 900.

3. **Youtube** - My entire career as a content creator, the reason you are reading this book at all, is because one Youtube page (GaryVee) taught me how to take my passion to social media and grow a following. And the same way that I learned how to build KetoSnackz in 2018, I am confident that anyone can find a Youtube channel that resonates with them and learn how to get healthy in 2022.

4. **Hobbies** - I moved to Texas as someone who went running 4-5x per week but eventually stopped because I couldn't keep up the habit in the summer heat. A year and a half had passed and I really missed going for my runs. So rather than go at it alone, I found a running group on the app MEETUP. It was amazing how easy it was to get back into the habit when I was around other people who were doing it too! I felt like I was part of a community and they were holding me accountable. Eventually I stopped going due to a schedule conflict but I kept up the habit of going running. As I write this I can proudly say I went for a 5 mile run in 102°F weather yesterday!

Chapter 16: Last Resort

Tracking calories can either be really helpful or really harmful depending on how much food anxiety you have. However, research shows that this is the single most beneficial habit to adopt if you want guaranteed results. And calorie counting on a low carb diet will be a totally different experience than calorie counting on a diet filled with sugar and bread. This is because you won't be on a blood sugar roller coaster all day or dealing with the whacked out hunger hormones that you're used to. It is much easier than you think it will be, I promise.

As you know from reading my story, I was very opposed to counting calories when I first got started on my keto journey. I also have generally been able to maintain a healthy weight just from keto for the past 5 years. So this approach was never necessary for me. The reason I gave it a try is due to the fact that I got a little too flirty with cheat days during pregnancy, gained 15 lbs and then saw it as an opportunity to find out if calorie counting really worked. It turns out that it does, especially when paired with keto.

The first thing you want to do is find a calorie calculator, then enter your information and your goals and that will give you a limit to stay under. However, it's very important that you don't set unrealistic goals. For example; the goal of losing 3 lbs per week gave me a ridiculously low calorie limit that I knew I would never be able to sustain. But the limit it gave me for the goal of losing ½ lb per week was only a 250 calorie deficit each day, which meant if I picked the right foods I never had to go to bed hungry.

But what if you have 150 lbs to lose and don't want to spend the next 3 years dieting? The first thing to realize is that in order to keep the weight off, you will have to spend the rest of your life doing some form of dieting. Not in the traditional calorie counting sense. Maybe not even by doing keto for the rest of your life either. But it is simply a fact that we all will have to be mindful of the foods we eat and in some cases even the portion sizes of those foods for the rest of our lives.

The next thing to realize is that a severely overweight person will lose weight much faster than a slightly overweight person. So don't get overwhelmed by the weekly goal that the app tells you. Lastly, the more overweight you are, the less fat you need to consume in order to live a low carb, low calorie lifestyle while still burning fat for fuel. Because your body just has more of it to tap into!

Here are some strategies that helped me on my calorie counting journey:

Guesstimating -

If the first week feels confusing and overwhelming there is nothing wrong with guesstimating. You simply want to make it a habit to log everything you eat. Even using a food diary and writing down what you ate is a good start. You can get the food scale and start weighing everything later on. Just accept that like learning any new skill, it won't be a smooth process in the beginning.

Intuitive fasting -

Any form of fasting is going to be significantly easier when paired with keto because keto does a great job at making hunger feel less urgent. So as long as you are not actually hungry, skipping meals can be a game changer for maintaining a deficit. I like to call this strategy "Intuitive fasting". It is similar to intermittent fasting, which induces weight-loss for many people because they naturally end up eating less calories throughout the day, similar to how keto works. But instead of making sure to eat everything in a 6 or 8 hour window, I have the flexibility to just eat when I feel hungry. This works really well for me because I love eating late at night but I also don't want to miss out on the benefits of getting protein first thing in the morning. And who doesn't love a delicious coffee?! If I were intermittent fasting, I would have to pick one or the other.

Budgeting -

Another thing that made calorie counting easier for me was learning to treat my energy balance like a financial budget. For example; It is hard to afford that big vacation without saving. And it is equally hard to make room for that big dinner without removing the unnecessary calories throughout the day.

Volume eating -

This is easily the best way to sustain a calorie deficit. When you realize how many more calories a candy bar has than a full plate of chicken and vegetables it will blow your mind. Rather than taking a super high fat approach to your weight-loss journey, volume eating lets you use mostly protein, fiber and some healthy fats to fill up your plate while skipping the processed fats and carbs that add up way too fast. The key to succeed with volume eating is to eat tons of lean protein, find the vegetables that you actually enjoy without being drowned in ranch and source your fat from whole foods like avocado and eggs.

PART 4
WHAT TO EAT

So now you've learned that you basically just have to eat less carbs to live a Care Free Keto lifestyle, but you might be wondering what the heck is left to eat then? If I'm not having bagels for breakfast and pasta for dinner what am I going to have?! What do I buy at the grocery store? What about when I go out to eat? In this part of the book you will find a grocery list, a fast food guide and tips for dining out!

This part of the book isn't meant to be followed 100%. There are many foods you can eat that aren't listed and many foods you don't have to eat that are listed. Think of the information here as a reference guide.

Chapter 17: Groceries

Let's take a stroll through the grocery store!

Dairy:

Butter, ghee, blocks of cheese, cheese slices, cheese sticks, shredded cheese, grated cheese, cream cheese, cottage cheese, low carb yogurt, eggs, heavy cream, half n half, sugar free whipped cream, sour cream, buttermilk, whey-protein & queso.

What I buy:

Butter	All cooking at low to medium temperatures.
Eggs	Scrambled, over-easy or in baking recipes.
Shredded cheddar	Salads, cheese-shells or cheese chips.
Shredded Mozzarella	Pizza topping, fat-head dough or zucchini noodle spaghetti.
Sliced American	Bunless burgers or low-carb bread sandwiches.
Yogurt	Dessert with nut butter and / or chocolate collagen.
Block of Cream Cheese	Baking recipes, in stuffed chicken or spread on bacon.
Heavy Cream	Baking recipes or in coffee.
Sour Cream	Dipping sauces or Mexican recipes.
Buttermilk	Soaking chicken or home-made ranch.

Pro-tip:
Pro-tip: Certain dairy products can have WAY more carbs than others, so be mindful of how many carbs are in a serving & how many servings you will actually consume. For example; I rarely consume less than 3 servings of cheese at a time. So if I buy a bag of shredded cheese that has 4g of carbs per serving I could end up over-doing my carbs for the day without realizing it. I would be much better off finding a bag of cheese with 1g of carbs per serving and making sure to measure out a serving before eating it.

Meat:

Beef, Chicken, Pork, & Turkey.

What I buy:

Ground Beef	Bunless burgers, meat sauce or tacos.
Bacon	With eggs, bunless burgers or low-carb bread sandwiches
Ribeye Steak	Served with asparagus, mashed cauliflower or brussels sprouts.
Chicken Thighs	Baked with crispy skin, taco seasoned on the grill or air fried.
Chicken Breast	Stuffed chicken, breaded with pork rinds or slow cooked.
Deli Turkey	Lettuce wraps, low-carb bread sandwiches or snacking.
Pepperoni Slices	Pizza or topped with cream cheese & everything bagel.
Hot Italian Sausage	Stuffed sausage, pizza or in stuffed peppers.

Pro-tip:

Basically all meat is safe to consume on a keto diet. Just be extra careful with sweetened meats from the deli such as honey ham, meats that come breaded such as chicken nuggets and meats that come pre sauced.

Also;

You may notice that I am listing things such as "pizza" and "tacos" when referring to what I use certain ingredients for. Please note that I am referring to keto versions of these foods.

Vegetables:

Artichokes, arugula, asparagus, bok choy, broccoli, brussels sprouts, cabbage, carrots, cauliflower, celery, chard, collard greens, garlic, green beans, jalapeños, jicama, kale, lettuce, mushrooms, onions, okra, radishes, seaweed, spinach, swiss chard.

What I buy:

Asparagus	Served as a side with meat.
Broccoli	Casseroles, roasted or drowning in cheese.
Brussels Sprouts	Smashed & air fried until crispy with parmesan.
Cabbage	Cooked with sausage & alfredo sauce.
Cauliflower	Mashed, riced & roasted.
Romaine lettuce	Bunless burgers, low-carb sandwiches or lettuce wraps.
Onions	Burgers, pizza topping, low carb sandwiches or air fried into cheese crisps.

Pro tip:

Some people believe that the carbs from vegetables don't count, however this is not true if the goal is ketosis. While vegetables do have a low glycemic index, meaning they are typically less impactful on blood sugar than things like flour & sugar, they can still knock you out of ketosis if you over-do them.

Fruit:

Avocados, bell peppers, blackberries, blueberries, cucumbers, eggplant, lemon, lime, olives, pickles, peaches, pumpkin, raspberries, squash, strawberries, tomatoes, zucchini.

What I buy:

Avocados	Burgers, salads or guac.
Bell peppers	Stuffed peppers, stir-fry recipes or as a chip replacement.
Berries	Salad, dessert recipes or snacking.
Olives	Pizza, salad or snacking.
Pickles	Burgers, lettuce wraps or snacking.
Spaghetti squash	Pasta recipes.
Tomatoes	Used as burger buns, on salads or BLT's.
Zucchini	Spiralized into noodles or in stir-fry recipes

Pro tip:

The carbs from fruit can add fast so be very mindful about serving sizes.

Also;

If you are simply trying to improve your health without "ketosis" as a primary goal, it's important to remember that all fruit is healthy.

Fats & Oils:

Avocado oil, bacon grease, beef tallow, coconut oil, ghee, lard, macadamia nut oil, MCT oil, olive oil.

What I buy:

Avocado oil	High heat cooking.
Olive oil	Low / medium heat cooking or salad dressings.

Pro tip:

Technically more affordable options like canola & corn oil won't knock you out of ketosis, but I try to avoid them because they are inflammatory.

Nuts, Seeds & Nut Butter:

Almonds, almond butter, brazil nuts, cashews, chia seeds, flax seeds, hazelnuts, hemp seeds, peanuts, peanut butter, pecans, pecan butter, pili nuts, pili butter, pistachios, sunflower seeds, macadamia nuts, & walnuts.

What I buy:

Almonds	Snacking or salads
Peanuts	Snacking
Peanut butter	Baking recipes, snacking or fat bombs
Macadamia nuts	Snacking

Pro tip:

Nuts are very high in calories, so if the goal is weight loss I definitely recommend portioning your nuts.

Sauce:

Alfredo, buffalo sauce, blue cheese, sugar free BBQ, caesar, hot sauce, italian dressing, no sugar added ketchup, marinara, mayonnaise, mustard, hot mustard, dijon mustard, ranch, salsa, sriracha, tartar sauce.

What I buy:

Alfredo sauce	Pizza or zucchini noodle / spaghetti squash recipes.
Sugar free BBQ	Chicken wings, blackened chicken tenders or marinade.
Hot sauce	Chicken wings, pizza or Mexican recipes
No Sugar Added Ketchup	Eggs, chicken or burgers.
Marinara	Pizza, stuffed pepper recipes or zucchini noodle recipes.
Ranch	Salad, chicken or pizza.

Pro tip:

Products like marinara sauce may have upwards of 6g carbs per serving, so be mindful of serving size.

Also;

Products like ranch & mayo are loaded with vegetable oils. So if you are avoiding inflammatory ingredients that is something important to check for.

Beverages:

Coffee, diet soda, sparkling water, sparkling ice, unsweetened nut milk, unsweetened tea, gatorade zero, powerade zero, vitamin water zero, zevia, & sugar free energy drinks.

What I buy :

Coffee	With heavy cream, protein shakes or unsweetened almond milk.
Diet soda	With dinner while eating out.
Sparkling water	Throughout the day.
Unsweetened almond milk	In coffee.
Gatorade zero	Occasionally on a hot day.

Pro tip:

I primarily drink water, however if diet soda is the only thing keeping you on track, please don't feel guilty about it. You are much more likely to run into serious health issues from being overweight than you are from drinking diet soda. The studies that suggest that diet soda could be harmful are not representative of the way we consume diet soda, they were done on rats that were given large amounts equivalent to a 150-pound human drinking 35+ cans of diet soda per day.

Also;

Things like gatorade zero, powerade zero, etc. are not a sufficient source of electrolytes. I drink them for taste.

KETO Snacks & sweets:

When buying savory snacks I'm primarily focused on carb count and less focused on the ingredient label. However, I am ALWAYS looking at the net carb count and the ingredient label for sweets and sweeteners. There are certain sweeteners used in "keto" treats that raise your blood sugar and kick you out of ketosis. So be sure to check that none of the sweets or sweeteners you buy have maltitol, maltodextrin, or dextrose on the ingredient label.

What I buy :

Quest frosted cookies
Enlightened ice cream bars
Highkey Mini Chocolate Chip Cookies
Perfect Keto Mallow Munch Bars
Hilo Life Snacks Tortilla Style Chips
Parm Crisps

Pro tip:

These foods are extremely easy to overeat. So always measure out your portions and make sure you aren't eating them out of boredom. I have an ice cream bar every night because it keeps the carb cravings away, but I NEVER eat them for fun or to fill the void when I'm having a bad day.

Baking swaps:

Keto baking is a great way to satisfy your sweet tooth without spending a ton of money on prepackaged keto snacks. These are some ingredients I try to keep in the pantry!

Flour	Coconut Flour, Almond Flour & Lupin Flour.
Sugar	Allulose, Monk Fruit, Erythritol, Stevia & Sucralose.
Breading	Pork Rinds (blended), Nutritional Yeast, Almond Flour, Coconut Flour.
Corn starch	Xanthan Gum.
Baking chips	Lily's, Choc Zero & Bake Believe Chocolate Chips.
Vegetable oil	Avocado Oil, Coconut Oil & Butter.
Milk	Unsweetened Almond Milk, Fairlife Milk & Heavy Cream.

Pro tip:

Like I mentioned with the snacks & sweets section, please check the ingredient labels of your sweeteners. There are lots of sweeteners at the grocery that claim to be "stevia" but actually use maltodextrin and dextrose as the primary ingredient.

Alcohol:

Liquor - Basically all non-flavored liquors will be fine!

Hard seltzers - There are countless brands of hard seltzers with 0-3g of carbs per serving. There will probably be 10 new brands on the market by time you read this book.

Wine - Dry wine is typically the lowest in carbs. Sauvignon Blanc, Pinot Blanc, Pinot Grigio, Pinot Noir, & Merlot are some of the lowest carb options. Just be mindful

about how many grams of carbs your wine has and keep track of your servings!

Beer: (net carbs per serving):
Greens trailblazer (0.5g net carbs)
Budweiser select (1.9g net carbs)
Miller 64 (2.4g net carbs)
Corona Premier (2.6g net carbs)
Michelob Ultra (2.6g net carbs)
Miller lite (3.2 net carbs)
Busch light (3.2 net carbs)
Natural light (3.2 net carbs)

Chapter 18: Fast Food & Dining Out

McDonalds:

Steak, egg and cheese biscuit, no biscuit.

- Cals: 303
- Fat: 19g
- Protein: 29g
- Net Carbs: 4g

Bacon egg and cheese biscuit, no biscuit.

- Cals: 189
- Fat: 13g
- Protein: 14g
- Net Carbs: 4g

Sausage patty.

- Cals: 190
- Fat: 18g
- Protein: 7g
- Net Carbs: 1g

Bacon.

- Cals: 70
- Fat: 4.5g
- Protein: 5g
- Net Carbs: 1g

Steak patty.

- Cals: 130
- Fat: 10g
- Protein: 12g
- Net Carbs: 0g

Round egg.

- Cals: 70
- Fat: 5g
- Protein: 7g
- Net Carbs: 1g

Folded egg.

- Cals: 60
- Fat: 4g
- Protein: 6g
- Net Carbs: 2g

Plain McDouble no bun.

- Cals: 220
- Fat: 16g
- Protein: 17g
- Net Carbs: 3g

Plain bacon McDouble no bun.

- Cals: 290
- Fat: 21g
- Protein: 23g
- Net Carbs: 3g

Plain McDouble no bun, add Mac sauce shredded lettuce, onions, pickles.

- Cals: 317
- Fat: 25g
- Protein: 18g
- Net Carbs: 5g

Double Quarter Pounder with Cheese, no bun, no ketchup.

- Cals: 587
- Fat: 43g
- Protein: 45g
- Net Carbs: 5g

Mushroom and Swiss Burger, no bun.

- Cals: 450
- Fat: 34g
- Protein: 26g
- Net Carbs: 9g
- Fiber: 1g

Bacon Ranch Salad w/ grilled chicken, no dressing:

- Cals: 318
- Fat: 14g
- Protein: 42g
- Net Carbs: 6g

Side Salad, no dressing.

- Cals: 15
- Fat: 0g
- Protein: 1g
- Net Carbs: 2g
- Fiber: 1g

Plain Grilled Chicken sandwich, no bun.

- Cals: 130
- Fat: 2g
- Protein: 28g
- Net Carbs: 0g

Plain McChicken, no bun.

- Cals: 160
- Fat: 9g
- Protein: 9g
- Net Carbs: 9g
- Fiber: 1g

Bacon Ranch Salad w/ grilled chicken, no dressing:

- Cals: 318
- Fat: 14g
- Protein: 42g
- Net Carbs: 6g

Side Salad, no dressing.

- Cals: 15
- Fat: 0g
- Protein: 1g
- Net Carbs: 2g
- Fiber: 1g

Mac sauce.

- Cals: 90
- Fat: 9g
- Protein: 0g
- Net Carbs: 2g

Wendys:

Baconator, no bun, no ketchup:

- Cals: 772
- Fat: 60g
- Protein: 53g
- Net Carbs: 5g

Double Stack, no bun, no ketchup.

- Cals: 263
- Fat: 19g
- Protein: 20g
- Net Carbs: 3g

Beef patty.

- Cals: 240
- Fat: 16g
- Protein: 18g
- Net Carbs: 0g

Jr. Beef patty.

- Cals: 120
- Fat: 8g
- Protein: 10g
- Net Carbs: 0g

Grilled Chicken Breast, plain.

- Cals: 130
- Fat: 1.5g
- Protein: 27g
- Net Carbs: 3g

Bacon.

- Cals: 20
- Fat: 1.5g
- Protein: 2g
- Net Carbs: 0g

Side salad, no dressing.

- Cals: 25
- Fat: 0g
- Protein: 1g
- Net Carbs: 3g
- Fiber: 2g

Southwest Avocado Salad, Half.

- Cals: 310
- Fat: 21g
- Protein: 22g
- Net Carbs: 6g
- Fiber: 4g

Parmesan Caesar Chicken Salad, Half.

- Cals: 316
- Fat: 20g
- Protein: 29g
- Net Carbs: 5g
- Fiber: 4g

Chick Fil-A:

Cobb Salad, No Chicken:

- Cals: 290
- Fat: 17g
- Protein: 15g

- Net Carbs: 15g
- Fiber: 5g

Bacon, Egg, and Cheese Biscuit, No Biscuit

- Cals: 210
- Fat: 16g
- Protein: 19g
- Net Carbs: 3g
- Fiber: 0g
-

Grilled Nuggets, 12 piece.

- Cals: 210
- Fat: 5g
- Protein: 38g
- Net Carbs: 3g
- Fiber: 0g

Burger King:

Whopper with cheese, no bun:

- Cals: 510
- Fat: 42g
- Protein: 25g
- Net Carbs: 8g
- Fiber: 0g

Double Whopper no bun, ketchup, or onions:

- Cals: 880
- Fat: 71
- Protein: 60g
- Net Carbs: 2g
- Fiber: 0g

Bacon King Jr, no bun, no sauce:

- Cals: 440
- Fat: 37g
- Protein: 25g
- Net Carbs: 1g
- Fiber: 0g

Chicken Club Salad, grilled chicken:

- Cals: 610
- Fat: 41g
- Protein: 46g
- Net Carbs: 11g
- Fiber: 7g

Sausage, egg and cheese biscuit no biscuit:

- Cals: 280
- Fat: 24g
- Protein: 14g
- Net Carbs: 1g
- Fiber: 0g

Bacon, egg, and cheese biscuit, no biscuit.

- Cals: 150
- Fat: 12g
- Protein: 9g
- Net Carbs: 1g
- Fiber: 0g

Five Guys:

Bacon cheeseburger, no bun.

- Cals: 370

- Fat: 30g
- Protein: 24g
- Net Carbs: 0g
- Fiber: 0g

Bacon, 2 slices:

- Cals: 80
- Fat: 7g
- Protein: 4g
- Net Carbs: 0g
- Fiber: 0g

Beef patty:

- Cals: 220
- Fat: 17g
- Protein: 16g
- Net Carbs: 0g
- Fiber: 0g

Hot dog, no bun:

- Cals: 240
- Fat: 20g
- Protein: 11g
- Net Carbs: 2g
- Fiber: 0g

Cheese:

- Cals: 70
- Fat: 6g
- Protein: 4g
- Net Carbs: 0g
- Fiber: 0g

Jalapeno peppers:

- Cals: 3
- Fat: 0g

- Protein: 0g
- Net Carbs: 0.5g
- Fiber: 0g

Onions:

- Cals: 10
- Fat: 0g
- Protein: 0g
- Net Carbs: 2g
- Fiber: 0g

Lettuce:

- Cals: 4
- Fat: 0g
- Protein: 0g
- Net Carbs:
- 1g Fiber: 0g

Pickles:

- Cals: 4
- Fat: 0g
- Protein: 0g
- Net Carbs: 1g
- Fiber: 0g

Subway:

Ham protein bowl, no dressing.

- Cals: 170
- Fat: 5g
- Protein: 21g
- Net Carbs: 9g
- Fiber: 3g

Buffalo chicken protein

bowl.

- Cals: 370
- Fat: 20g
- Protein: 35g
- Net Carbs: 10g
- Fiber: 3g

Chicken bacon ranch protein bowl.

- Cals: 600
- Fat: 40g
- Protein: 52g
- Net Carbs: 9g
- Fiber: 3g
-

Cold cut protein bowl, no dressing.

- Cals: 260
- Fat: 16g
- Protein: 20g
- Net Carbs: 6g
- Fiber: 3g

Steak & cheese protein bowl, no dressing.

- Cals: 380
- Fat: 19g
- Protein: 42g
- Net Carbs: 8g
- Fiber: 4g

Bacon, 2 strips:

- Cals: 80
- Fat: 5g
- Protein: 6g

- Net Carbs: 1g
- Fiber: 0g

Breakfast sausage:

- Cals: 140
- Fat: 11g
- Protein: 10g
- Net Carbs: 1g
- Fiber: 0g

Egg patty:

- Cals: 120
- Fat: 7g
- Protein: 9g
- Net Carbs: 3g
- Fiber: 0g

KFC:

Grilled chicken breast.

- Cals: 210
- Fat: 7g
- Protein: 38g
- Net Carbs: 0g
- Fiber: 0g

Grilled chicken thigh.

- Cals: 150
- Fat: 9g
- Protein: 17g
- Net Carbs: 0g
- Fiber:0g

Grilled Chicken drumstick.

- Cals: 80

- Fat: 4g
- Protein: 13g
- Net Carbs: 0g
- Fiber: 0g

Green beans, side order.

- Cals: 25
- Fat: 0g
- Protein: 1g
- Net Carbs: 2g
- Fiber: 2g

Buttermilk ranch:

- Cals: 100
- Fat: 10g
- Protein: 0g
- Net Carbs: 2g
- Fiber: 0g

Popeyes:

Blackened Tenders, 3 piece.

- Cals: 170
- Fat: 2g
- Protein: 26g
- Net Carbs: 2g
- Fiber: 0g

Green beans, regular.

- Cals: 55
- Fat: 2g
- Protein: 3g
- Net Carbs: 5g
- Fiber: 2g

Panera:

Avocado, egg white & spinach, no bagel

- Cals: 160
- Fat: 11g
- Protein: 13g
- Net Carbs: 2g
- Fiber: 2g

Bacon turkey bravo, whole, no bread or sauce.

- Cals: 450
- Fat: 29g
- Protein: 39g
- Net Carbs: 8g
- Fiber: 1g

Greek salad, whole.

- Cals: 380 Fat: 36g Protein: 7g Net Carbs: 9g Fiber: 8g

Chicken caesar salad, whole, no croutons.

- Cals: 400
- Fat: 26g
- Protein: 32g
- Net Carbs: 7g
- Fiber: 10g

Green goddess chicken cobb salad, whole.

- Cals: 500
- Fat: 30g
- Protein: 42g
- Net Carbs: 10g

- Fiber: 7g

Panda Express:

Grilled teriyaki chicken.

- Cals: 300
- Fat: 13g
- Protein: 36g
- Net Carbs: 8g Fiber: 0g

String bean chicken breast.

- Cals: 190
- Fat: 9g
- Protein: 14g
- Net Carbs: 9g Fiber: 4g

Black pepper angus steak.

- Cals: 180
- Fat: 7g
- Protein: 19g
- Net Carbs: 9g Fiber: 1g

Kung pao chicken.

- Cals: 290
- Fat: 19g
- Protein: 16g
- Net Carbs: 12g Fiber: 3g

Firecracker shrimp.

- Cals: 110
- Fat: 4g
- Protein: 11g
- Net Carbs: 6g Fiber: 1g

Broccoli beef.

- Cals: 150

- Fat: 7g
- Protein: 9g
- Net Carbs: 11g Fiber: 3g

Super greens.

- Cals: 90
- Fat: 3g
- Protein: 6g
- Net Carbs: 5g
- Fiber: 5g

Jersey Mikes:

Original italian, in a tub.

- Cals: 380
- Fat: 21g
- Protein: 34g
- Net Carbs: 12g
- Fiber: 1g

California club, in a tub.

- Cals: 420
- Fat: 26g
- Protein: 35g
- Net Carbs: 7g
- Fiber: 5g

Chipotle turkey, in a tub.

- Cals: 530
- Fat: 42g Protein: 27g
- Net Carbs: 11g
- Fiber: 1g

Chicken philly, in a tub.

- Cals: 400

- Fat: 21g
- Protein: 37g
- Net Carbs: 15g Fiber: 1g

Steak philly, in a tub.

- Cals: 440
- Fat: 27g
- Protein: 35g
- Net Carbs: 13g
- Fiber: 1g

Big kahuna, in a tub.

- Cals: 490
- Fat: 31g
- Protein: 39g
- Net Carbs: 14g
- Fiber: 1g

Taco Bell:

Chicken Power Bowl, no beans or rice.

- Cals: 240
- Fat: 14g
- Protein: 21g
- Net Carbs: 4g
- Fiber: 3g

Steak power bowl, no beans or rice.

- Cals: 250
- Fat: 16g
- Protein: 20g
- Net Carbs: 6g
- Fiber: 2g

Beefy 5-layer burrito, no shell.

- Cals: 200
- Fat: 11g
- Protein: 10g
- Net Carbs: 10g
- Fiber: 6g

Chicken Quesadilla, no shell.

- Cals: 310
- Fat: 21g
- Protein: 22g
- Net Carbs: 3g
- Fiber: 2g

DINING OUT:

This is a quick reference guide based on what I order. One thing to remember is that marinades & sauces can bring the carb count of something up pretty high. So be sure to look up the nutrition facts for the specific restaurant you're at before ordering something that's saucy or glazed & decide if it will work for you.

Steakhouse:

What I order: Ribeye & loaded broccoli

Any combination of steak and vegetables is a great choice when dining at a steakhouse. They should have grilled chicken or bunless burgers on the menu too. Just be sure to avoid potatoes, sweet potatoes and breaded vegetables. Asking for loaded vegetables is a great choice because they put the sour cream, cheese & bacon from a loaded baked potato on your vegetables.

Chinese:

What I order: Kung Pao Chicken, no rice & extra vegetables

My favorite Chinese dish when I first started living a low carb lifestyle was beef and broccoli, but I quickly realized the sauce is very sugary. So be careful to check that specific restaurant's nutrition info if you want beef and broccoli. Other options are stir fried chicken, beef or shrimp with no sauce & a side of veggies.

Japanese:

What I order: Philadelphia roll no rice

Depending on the restaurant, you may be able to ask for a sushi roll without rice. However, one thing to consider if you go this route is that even without rice, breaded options like shrimp tempura will have a higher carb count than your typical roll with sashimi. Also, miso soup & steamed veggies are two of my favorite appetizers that are low in carbs.

Italian:

What I order: Chicken Alfredo, replace the noodles with broccoli

One of the best tips for Italian restaurants is to order the pasta dish of your choice and ask them to swap out the noodles for vegetables. You can usually find some sort of grilled meat or fish entree with veggies as well. Caesar salad with no croutons is a great appetizer.

BBQ:

What I order: Brisket, extra pickles & onions on the side with a serving of green beans

BBQ restaurants are great because most of the meat options are keto-friendly as long as you avoid the sauce.

Pro tip: Bring your own sugar free bbq sauce.

Sea Food:

What I order: Grilled salmon with a side of vegetables & scallops or shrimp

Salmon, grilled shrimp, lobster, scallops & crab legs are all great options. You can often order steak at Sea Food restaurants too which is a great choice.

Sports bar:

What I order: 10 hot wings with a side house salad & ranch

Sports bars and casual restaurants that serve wings are my favorite. Dry rub, naked, buffalo & hot wings are generally pretty low in carbs as long as they aren't breaded. Swap out the sides with a side salad or ask for extra carrots and celery. You can also get bunless burgers and grilled chicken salads.

Mexican:

What I order: Steak fajitas with no rice, beans or tortillas

Other options are taco salads with no rice or beans, grilled chicken with veggies and even stuffed peppers. If you can't resist the chips, ask for raw bell pepper slices and order a side of queso or guacamole! You can also bring your own pork rinds.

Chapter 19: Meal Plans

This is an adjustable 14-day plan that lets you alter the serving sizes based on your goals and lifestyle because an active male who weighs 250 pounds will need much larger portions to feel satisfied than a sedentary woman who weighs 165 lbs.

You can take two approaches to these meal plans -

Approach 1: Put your faith in keto and listen to your body

This is the approach that helped me get to a healthy weight and maintain it for 5 years. Because as discussed previously, keto does a great job at regulating your appetite and naturally putting you in a deficit. What you want to do with this approach is look at the meal plans and loosely follow them based on your hunger levels.

For example; The first lunch is "beef patties, with cheese, onions, pickles & mustard". But, what if you're a busy mom with 2 toddlers and you don't typically want a big lunch? Or what if keto has reduced your appetite to the point of not being hungry in the middle of the day? If that's the case you can either skip lunch and refer to the snack ideas or simply not eat at all if you don't want to. Because you are not going to speed up weight-loss by eating more than you are hungry for.

Approach 2: Calorie deficit

While this isn't the most Care Free approach, calorie counting can be powerful and sometimes even necessary for people who aren't seeing results. If you do prefer this approach you simply want to assess how hungry you are during each part of the day and then determine your portion sizes for each meal based on that.

Day 1:

Breakfast	Eggs cooked in butter with bacon
Lunch	2-4 beef patties with cheese, onions, pickles & mustard. Side salad, no croutons
Dinner	Zucchini Noodle Spaghetti with mozzarella, ground beef & marinara sauce
Dessert	Small serving of berries with sugar free whipped cream

Day 2:

Breakfast	Smoothie with protein powder, unsweetened almond milk, blueberries, peanut butter & ice
Lunch	Chicken caesar salad
Dinner	NY Strip steak & Mashed cauliflower

Day 3:

Breakfast	Rotisserie chicken with ranch
Snack	String cheese, Sugar free beef jerky & Green olives
Lunch -	Blackened chicken tenders, Bell pepper with cream cheese & everything bagel seasoning
Dinner	Chili lime salmon bites & Roasted broccoli

Day 4:

Breakfast	Tuna salad with pork rinds or veggies for dipping
Snack	Flavored almonds
Lunch	Chicken crust pizza
Dinner	Garlic butter steak bites & ½ avocado

Day 5:

Breakfast	Turkey roll up with cheese, lettuce, mayo & cucumber slices & ranch
Lunch	Zero carb chicken nuggets
Dinner	Cream cheese stuffed chicken with spinach
Dessert	No sugar added yogurt with almond butter

Day 6:

Breakfast	3-6 eggs with sliced ham & american cheese
Lunch	Pork chops with ranch & Roasted asparagus
Snack	Macadamia nuts
Dinner	Crispy skin chicken thighs & ½ avocado

Day 7:

Breakfast	Philly cheesesteak stuffed bell peppers
Lunch	Cobb salad
Dinner	Flank steak & Loaded broccoli
Snack	Cucumber with ranch
Dessert	Spoonful of peanut butter

Day 8:

Breakfast	Cheese shell wrap with eggs, bacon & guac
Lunch	Grilled chicken with alfredo sauce & hearts of palm noodles
Snack	Tuna salad with celery
Dinner	Buffalo chicken stuffed poblano pepper

Day 9:

Breakfast	Lettuce boat BLT
Lunch	Pork rind crusted chicken & Creamed spinach
Dinner	Taco salad

Day 10:

Breakfast	Coffee with protein shake
Lunch	Chicken bacon ranch skewers
Dinner	Ribeye steak & Garlic parmesan green beans

Day 11:

Breakfast	Ham wrapped egg bites
Lunch	Ground beef with marinara sauce
Dinner	Pork tenderloin & Roasted radishes

Day 12:

Breakfast	Deviled eggs
Lunch	Deli meat roll-up with cheese, lettuce, bacon & mayo
Dinner	Nutritional yeast crusted chicken cordon bleu & Prosciutto wrapped asparagus

Day 13:

Breakfast	Rotisserie chicken with ranch & Small serving of pistachios
Lunch	Pulled pork with sugar free BBQ sauce & Jalapeno poppers
Dinner	Carne Asada with cauliflower rice

Day 14:

Breakfast	No sugar added yogurt & Spoonful of nut butter
Snack	Flavored almonds & Beef jerky
Lunch	Blackened tenders & ½ avocado
Dinner	Low carb tortilla pizza

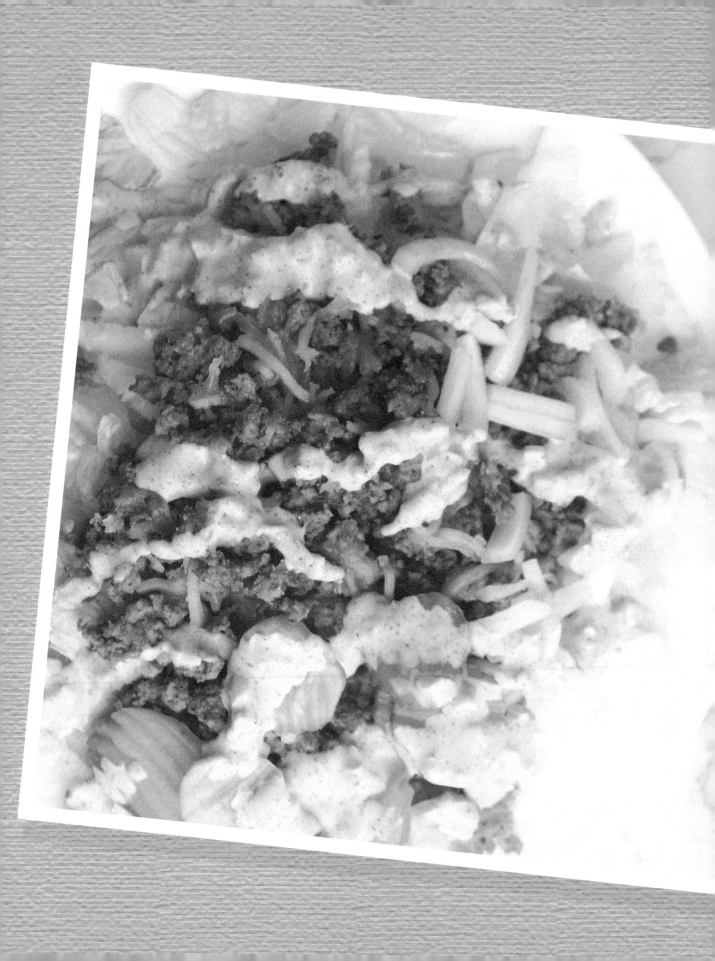

Meals

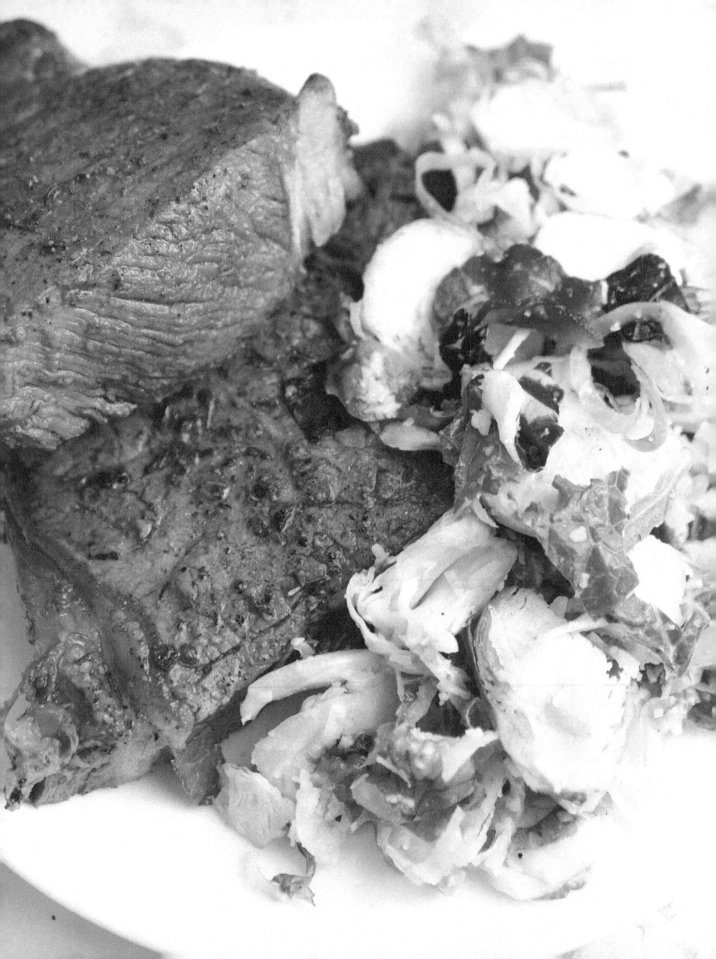

Air Fried Steak

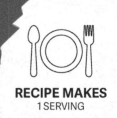

RECIPE MAKES
1 SERVING

MACROS

🔥 **CAL: 658**   🪔 **FAT: 41G**   🍳 **PROTEIN: 67G**

🌾 **TOTAL CARBS: 0G**   🍃 **FIBER: 0G**   🌾 **NET CARBS: 0G**

INGREDIENTS

- 8 oz steak (I prefer strip or ribeye)
- 1 tbsp butter
- 1 tbsp olive oil
- 1/8 tsp thyme
- 1/8 tsp oregano
- 1/2 tsp parsley
- Salt & pepper to taste

INSTRUCTIONS

1. Let steak sit until room temperature, about 30 mins.
2. Rub both sides of the steak with olive oil, thyme, oregano, salt & pepper.
3. Add to the air fryer at 400F for 5 minutes
4. Flip steak and put back in for 5 more minutes.
5. Mix your butter with the parsley and melt in the microwave.
6. When steak is finished, drizzle with the butter, let rest for 10 minutes and enjoy!

Notes:

This is for a 1 inch thick medium rare steak. For medium, cook 6 minutes on each side. For medium well, cook 7 minutes on each side.

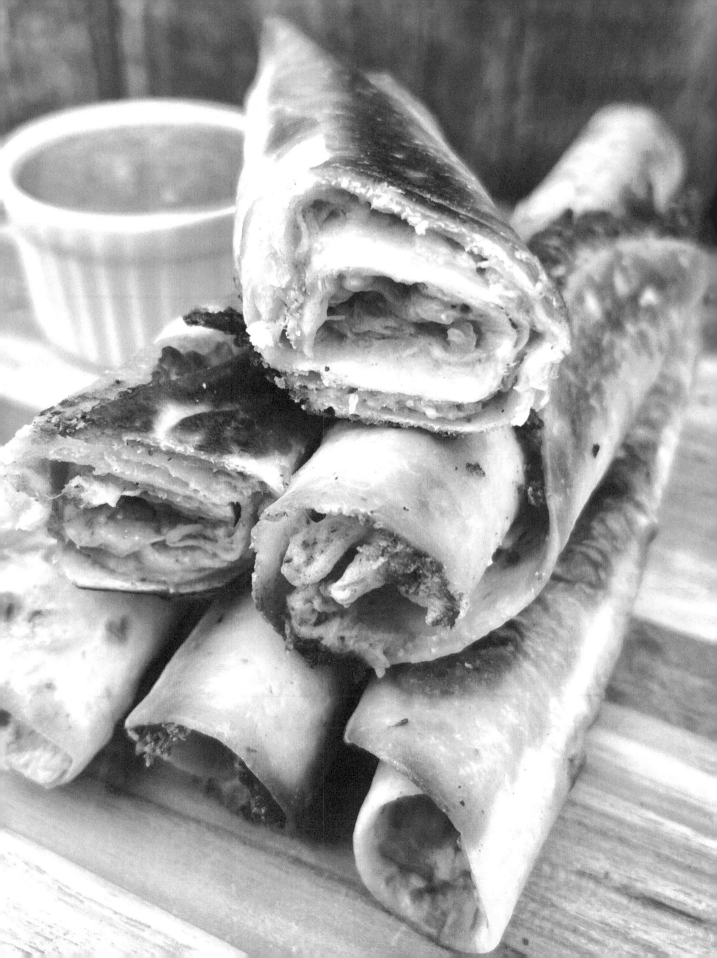

Buffalo Chicken Taquitos

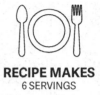

RECIPE MAKES
6 SERVINGS

MACROS

🔥 **CAL: 388**   🫗 **FAT: 27G**   🥚 **PROTEIN: 18G**

🌾 **TOTAL CARBS: 15G**   🍃 **FIBER: 10G**   🌾 **NET CARBS: 5G**

INGREDIENTS

- 4 low carb tortillas
- 1.5 cups shredded rotisserie chicken
- 1/4 cup Buffalo sauce
- 1/4 cup ranch dressing
- 1/4 cup shredded cheddar
- 4 oz cream cheese
- Oil for frying

INSTRUCTIONS

1. Preheat oven to 350F.
2. In a baking dish combine your chicken with the cream cheese, Buffalo sauce, ranch, & shredded cheddar.
3. Bake for 20 minutes.
4. Add to your tortillas and roll them up tightly.
5. Fry in oil until golden brown and crispy!
6. Remove from oil and place on paper towels, let cool, & enjoy!

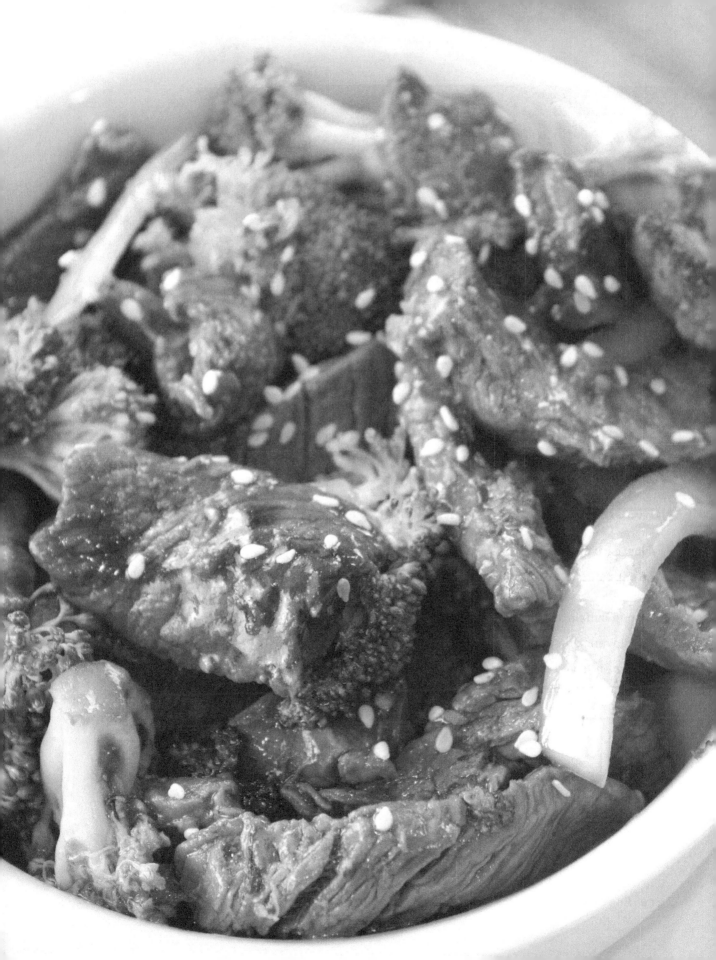

Beef & Broccoli

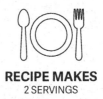

RECIPE MAKES
2 SERVINGS

MACROS

🔥 **CAL: 454**   🫗 **FAT: 30G**   🥑 **PROTEIN: 40G**

🌾 **TOTAL CARBS: 8G**   🍃 **FIBER: 2.5G**   **NET CARBS: 5.5G**

INGREDIENTS

- 12 oz thinly sliced beef, sirloin or tenderloin
- 2 cups chopped broccoli
- 1/4 cup soy sauce
- 2 tbsp beef broth
- 2 tbsp avocado oil
- 1-2 tbsp sweetener
- 2 tsp minced garlic
- 1/2 tsp ground ginger
- 1/4 tsp xanthan gum

INSTRUCTIONS

1. Slice your beef into bite sized strips.
2. Add skillet to stove on medium heat & cook the beef in avocado oil until browned, remove from skillet and set aside.
3. Reduce heat to medium low and cook the broccoli until tender.
4. Mix in the rest of your ingredients and stir until it thickens.
5. Remove from heat, & enjoy!

Note:

During step 4, it helps to sprinkle in your xanthan gum while stirring to avoid clumping.

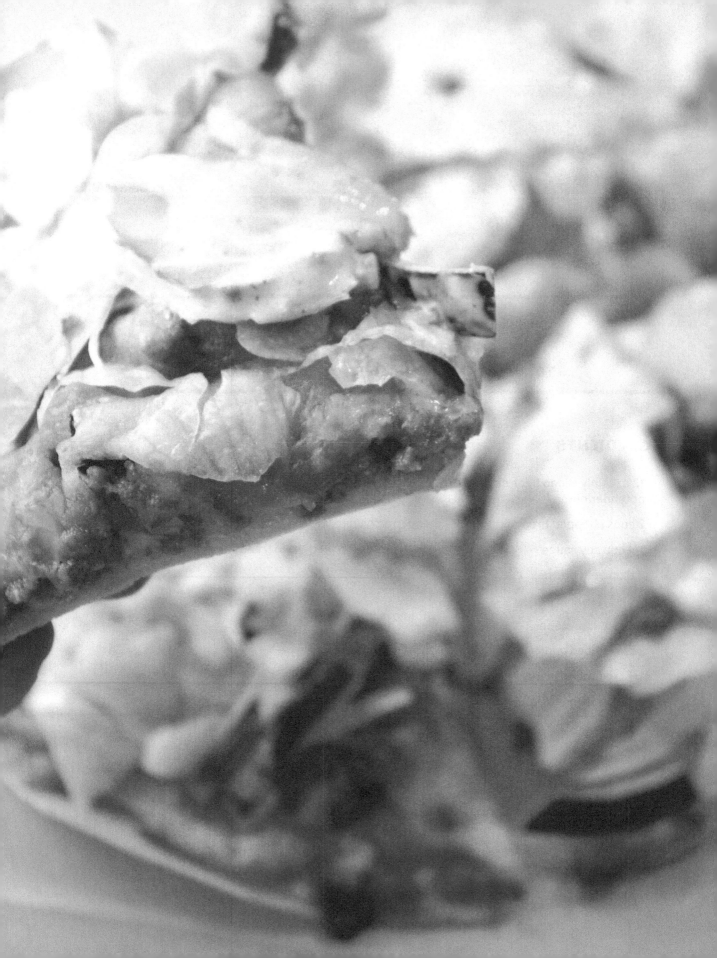

Big Mac Pizza

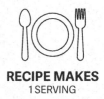

RECIPE MAKES
1 SERVING

MACROS

 CAL: 861   FAT: 67G   PROTEIN: 53G
 TOTAL CARBS: 24G   FIBER: 17G   NET CARBS: 7G

INGREDIENTS

- Low carb tortilla
- 1 cup fully cooked beef
- 1/2 cup shredded cheddar
- 1/4 cup shredded mozzarella
- 1/4 cup shredded lettuce
- 1/3 cup mac sauce (recipe on next page)
- 2 tbsp pickles
- 2 tbsp onions

INSTRUCTIONS

1. Broil your tortilla for 1-2 minutes. Remove and add to a baking sheet.

2. Spread on the mac sauce. Top with beef, onions, & cheese.

3. Bake at 400F for 10 minutes.

4. Take out, add lettuce, pickles, more onions & more mac sauce.

5. Enjoy!

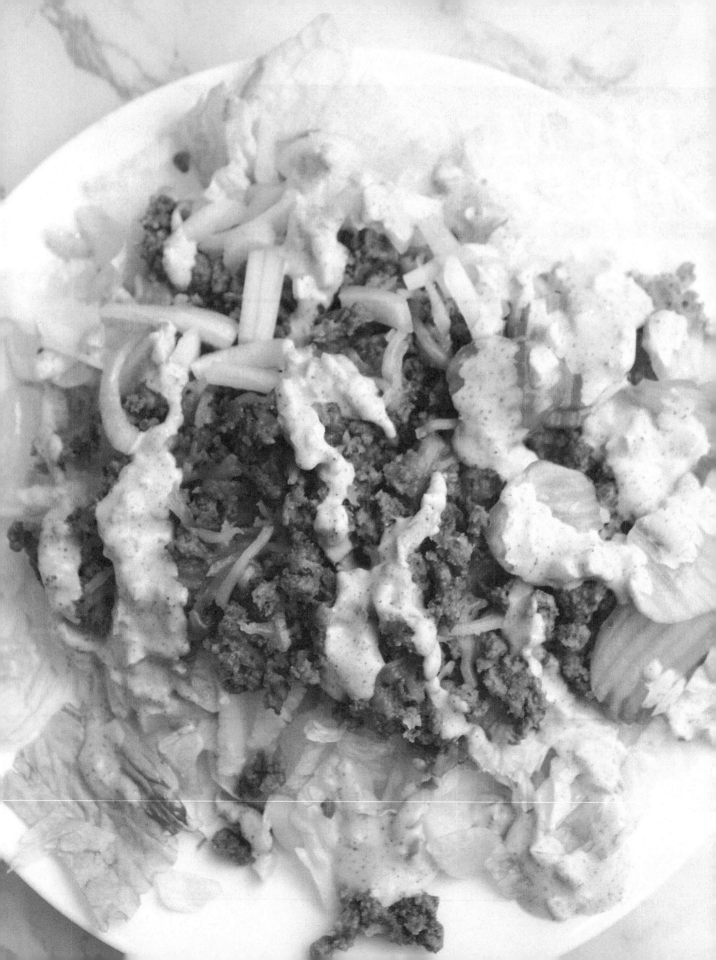

Big Mac Salad

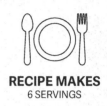

RECIPE MAKES
6 SERVINGS

MACROS

🔥 **CAL: 200**   🌢 **FAT: 22G**   🫘 **PROTEIN: 0G**

🌾 **TOTAL CARBS: 0.3G**   🍃 **FIBER: 0G**   🌾 **NET CARBS: 0.3G**

INGREDIENTS

For the Sauce:

- 3/4 cup mayonnaise
- 1 tbsp mustard
- 2 tbsp chopped dill pickles
- 1 tbsp white vinegar
- 1 tbsp chopped onions
- 2 tsp sweetener
- 1/2 tsp smoked paprika

For the salad:

- 2 cups romaine lettuce
- 1/4 lb ground beef (fully cooked & seasoned)
- 1/4 cup shredded cheddar cheese
- 2 tbsp chopped pickles
- 2 tbsp chopped onions
- 2-3 tbsp Mac Sauce
- Salt & pepper to taste

INSTRUCTIONS

For the Sauce:

1. Mix all ingredients well.
2. Add to squirt bottle or air tight container and use as needed.

For the salad:

1. Toss all ingredients in a large bowl & enjoy!

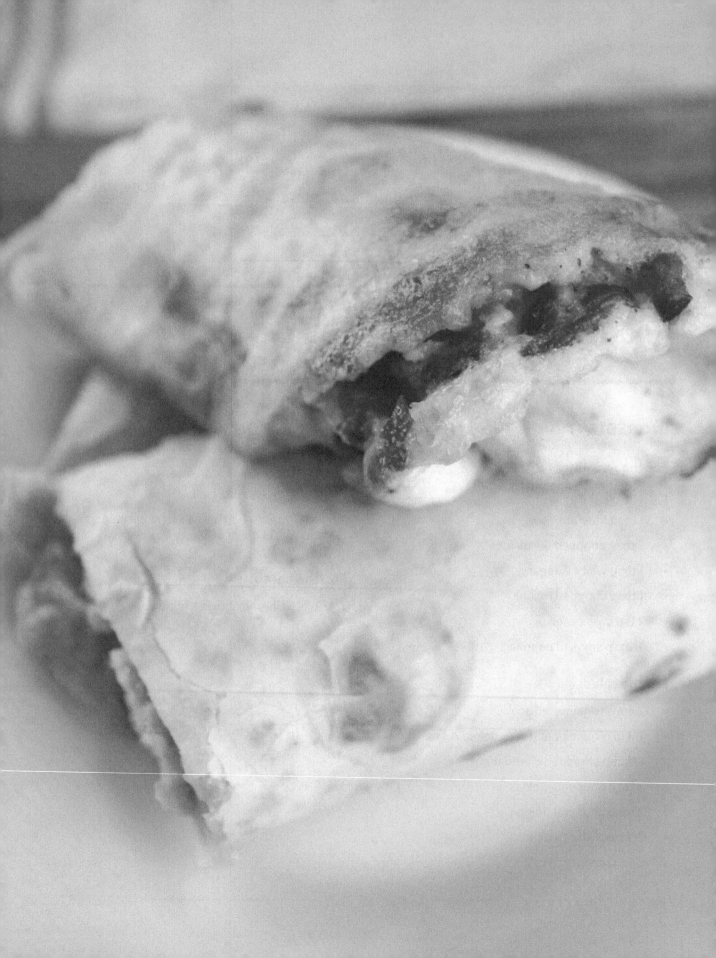

Breakfast Skillet Wrap

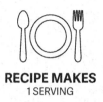

RECIPE MAKES
1 SERVING

MACROS

🔥 **CAL: 559**   💧 **FAT: 47G**   🫘 **PROTEIN: 27G**

🌾 **TOTAL CARBS: 21G**   🍃 **FIBER: 15G**   🌾 **NET CARBS: 6G**

INGREDIENTS

- 2 tbsp butter
- 2 eggs whisked
- 1/4 cup shredded cheddar cheese
- 2 slices bacon, cooked & crumbled
- Low carb tortilla, 8-inch

INSTRUCTIONS

1. Add your butter to a pan on medium low heat, add your eggs, cheese & bacon.

2. Top with tortilla, once the cheese sticks to the tortilla, flip, roll it up, & enjoy!

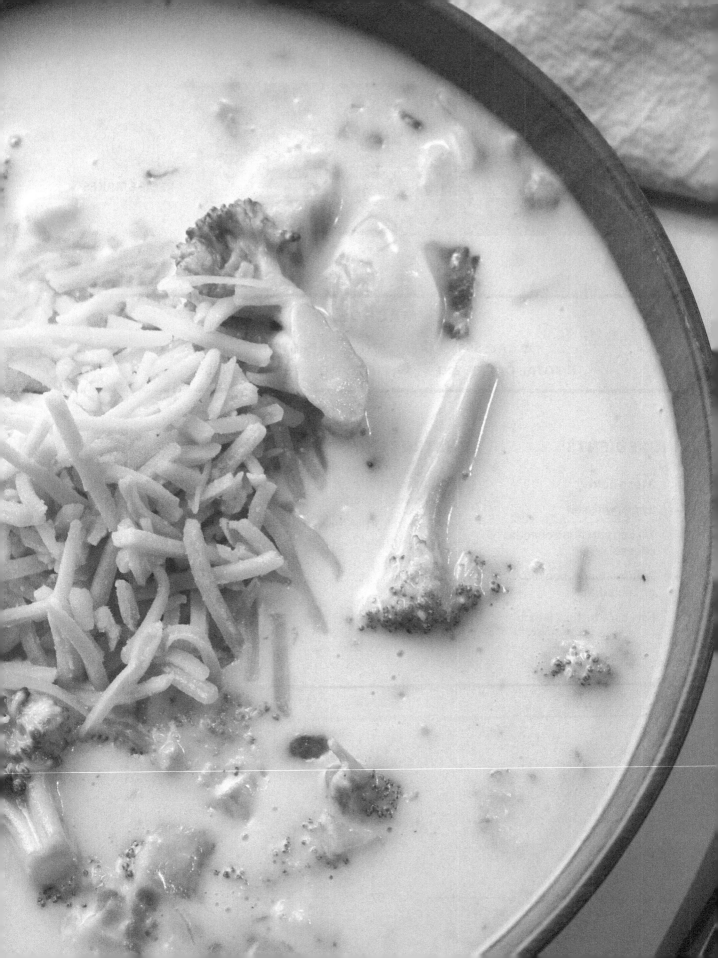

Broccoli Cheddar Soup

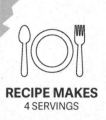

RECIPE MAKES
4 SERVINGS

MACROS

🔥 CAL: 417   🥑 FAT: 36G   🍳 PROTEIN: 19G

🌾 TOTAL CARBS: 8G   🍃 FIBER: 2G   🌾 NET CARBS: 6G

INGREDIENTS

- 1 medium head of broccoli florets
- 2 cups shredded cheddar cheese
- 1/2 cup heavy cream
- 1/2 cup bacon crumbles
- 1.5 cups chicken broth
- 1/2 onion, chopped
- 2 tbsp butter
- 1 clove garlic, minced
- Salt & pepper

INSTRUCTIONS

1. Melt your butter in a large saucepan over medium heat. Add your garlic, onion, salt & pepper and stir until the onions are translucent.

2. Add your chicken broth, cream, cheddar. Whisk until cheddar melts.

3. Add your broccoli & bacon and lower heat to simmer.

4. Stir until broccoli becomes tender.

5. Serve topped with more cheddar & enjoy!

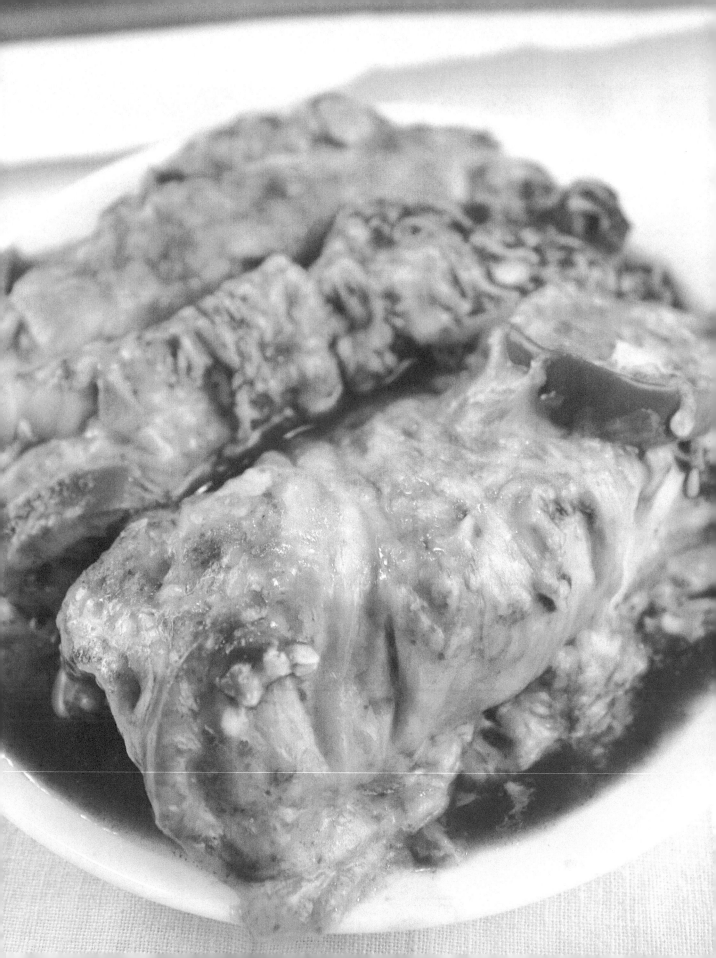

Cabbage Enchiladas

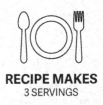

RECIPE MAKES
3 SERVINGS

MACROS

🔥 **CAL: 325**   💧 **FAT: 21G**   🥩 **PROTEIN: 27G**

🌾 **TOTAL CARBS: 9G**   🍃 **FIBER: 1G**   🌾 **NET CARBS: 8G**

INGREDIENTS

- 6 cabbage leaves
- 1/2 cup of enchilada sauce
- 1 cup shredded Mexican cheese
- Jalapeños for topping

Filling ingredients:

- 1 cup diced or shredded chicken, fully cooked
- 1/4 cup enchilada sauce
- 1/2 cup shredded Mexican cheese
- Seasonings of choice

INSTRUCTIONS

1. Preheat the oven to 350F.
2. Blanch cabbage leaves.
3. Mix chicken filling ingredients in a bowl.
4. Flatten cabbage leaves and scoop some chicken mix into them.
5. Roll them up and add to a baking dish.
6. Cover with the enchilada sauce & cheese.
7. Bake covered for 20 minutes. Remove cover & broil for 2-3 minutes,
8. Take out, let cool, & enjoy!

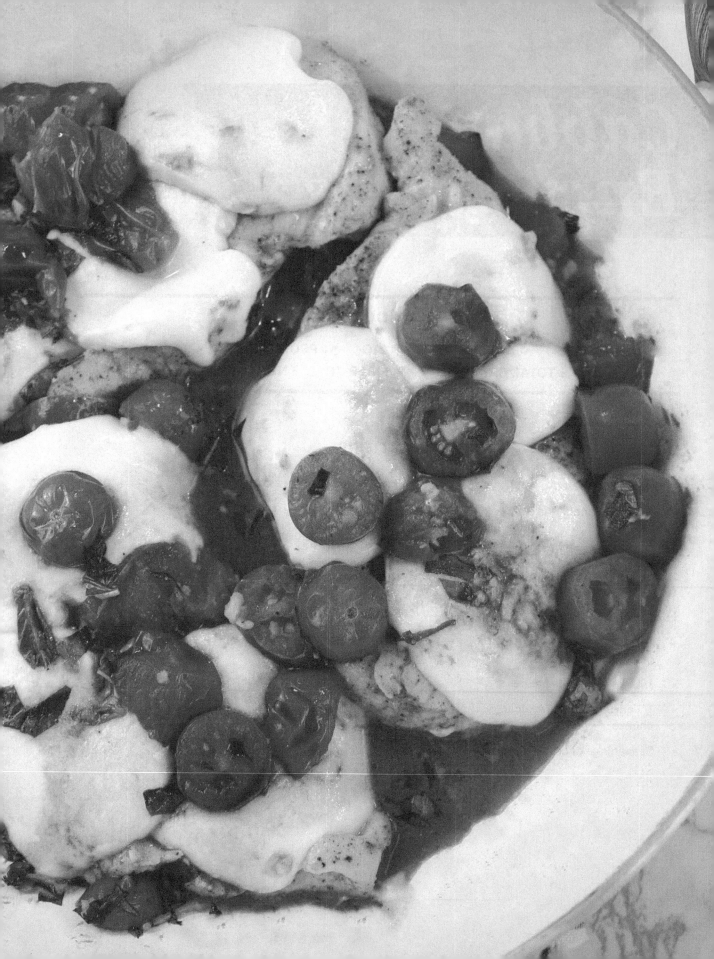

Caprese Chicken

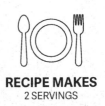

RECIPE MAKES
2 SERVINGS

MACROS

🔥 CAL: 356   💧 FAT: 23.5G   🍳 PROTEIN: 33G

🌾 TOTAL CARBS: 69G   🍃 FIBER: 1.8G   🌾 NET CARBS: 4.2G

INGREDIENTS

- 2 thinly sliced chicken breasts
- 4 oz fresh mozzarella, sliced
- 1 pint cherry tomatoes
- 2 tbsp fresh basil, chopped
- 2 tbsp olive oil
- 1 garlic clove, minced
- Salt & pepper
- Balsamic vinegar

INSTRUCTIONS

1. Slice chicken in half and add salt & pepper to both sides.

2. Add to a pan over medium high heat with 1 tbsp of oil and cook for 3-4 minutes on each side. When fully cooked, set aside and cover with foil.

3. Add the rest of your oil and the garlic to your pan and cook for 1 minute.

4. Add the tomatoes and continue sautéing until they begin to wrinkle.

5. Stir in your basil and add your chicken back to the pan.

6. Mix around, top with your fresh mozzarella, and cover until the cheese melts.

7. Drizzle with balsamic vinegar and enjoy!

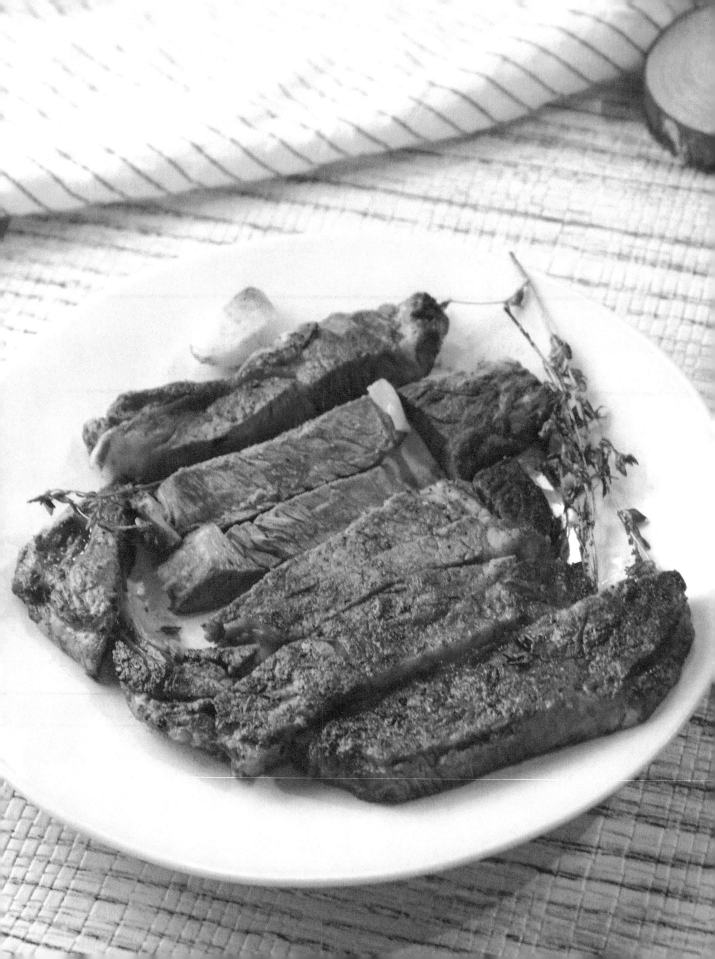

Cast Iron Ribeye

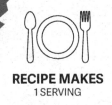

RECIPE MAKES
1 SERVING

MACROS

🔥 **CAL: 980** 🌢 **FAT: 61G** 🫛 **PROTEIN: 100G**
🌾 **TOTAL CARBS: 0G** 🍃 **FIBER:0G** 🌾 **NET CARBS: 0G**

INGREDIENTS

- 12 oz ribeye steak
- 2 tbsp oil
- 3 tbsp butter
- 4 garlic cloves
- 1/4 cup fresh thyme (optional)
- Salt & pepper

INSTRUCTIONS

1. Add salt and pepper to the steak and let rest at room temperature for 20 minutes.

2. Add oil to your cast iron over high heat & sear the steak on each side flipping every minute.

3. Add your garlic cloves and continue flipping each minute.

4. Add the butter & thyme and baste each side of the steak with the melted butter.

5. Remove from heat, let rest for 10 minutes, & enjoy!

Notes:

For a medium steak, flip every 2 minutes. For medium well, flip every 3 minutes.

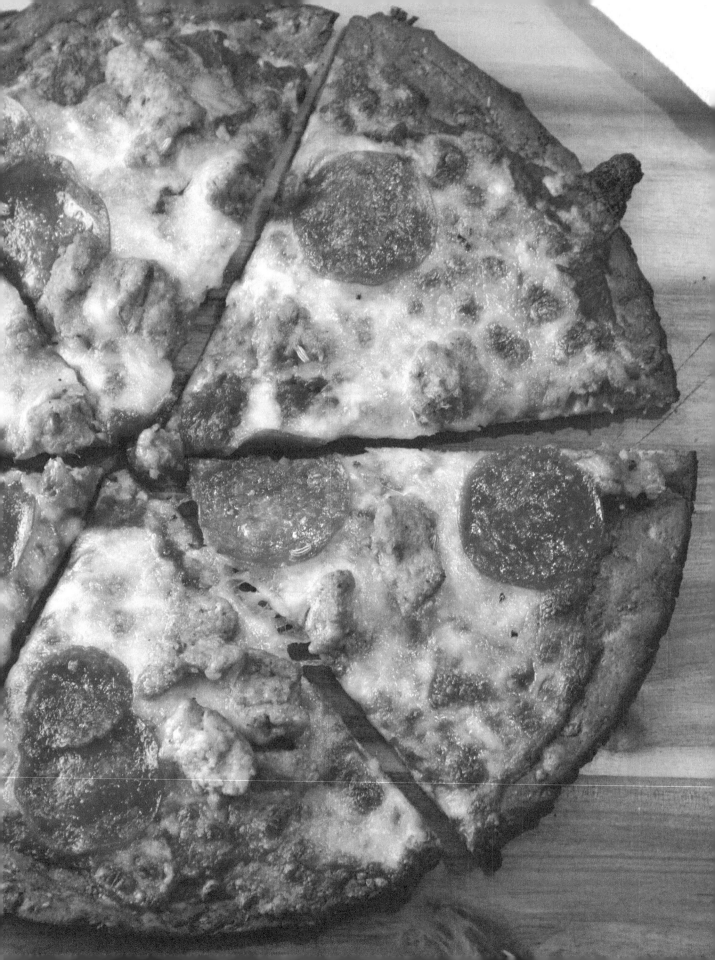

Cauliflower Crust Pizza

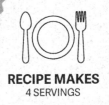

RECIPE MAKES
4 SERVINGS

MACROS (for crust only)

🔥 **CAL: 99**   💧 **FAT: 4G**   🍳 **PROTEIN: 9G**

🌾 **TOTAL CARBS: 9G**   🍃 **FIBER: 4G**   🌾 **NET CARBS: 5G**

INGREDIENTS

- 1.5 lbs cauliflower florets
- 1/2 cup shredded mozzarella
- 1 egg, beaten
- 1 tsp Italian seasoning
- Salt & pepper
- Toppings of your choice

INSTRUCTIONS

1. Preheat the oven to 400F.

2. Blend your cauliflower florets until riced.

3. Microwave for 4-5 minutes.

4. Drain all moisture with a cheesecloth.

5. Add to a mixing bowl with your cheese, egg, and seasoning.

6. On a parchment lined baking sheet shape the dough into a circle around 9 inches in diameter.

7. Bake for 20 minutes, flip, and put back in for 5-10 more minutes.

8. Add your toppings and place back in for 10 minutes.

9. Take out, let cool, and enjoy!

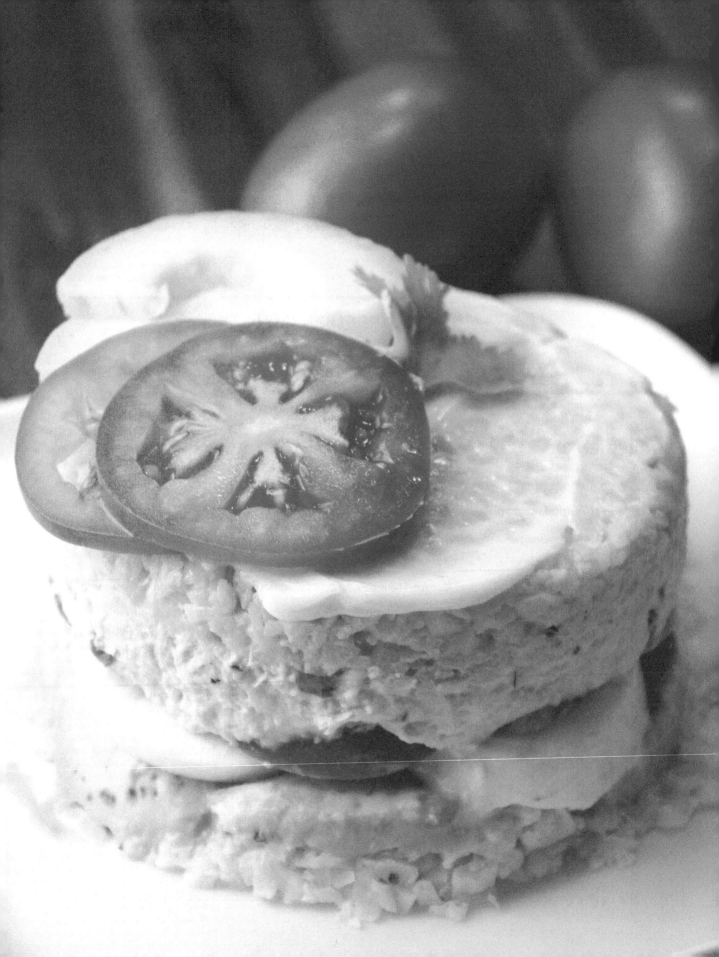

Causa Rellena

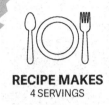

RECIPE MAKES
4 SERVINGS

MACROS (for crust only)

🔥 **CAL: 185G**   💧 **FAT: 12G**   🍳 **PROTEIN: 13G**

🌾 **TOTAL CARBS: 11.5G**   🍃 **FIBER: 5.6G**   🌾 **NET CARBS: 5.9G**

INGREDIENTS

- 1 lb riced cauliflower
- 1.5 tablespoon yellow pepper paste
- 1 tbsp fresh lime juice
- Salt & pepper to taste

Tuna Salad:

- 1 can of albacore tuna (in water)
- 1/4 finely chopped red onion
- 1 tbsp minced cilantro
- 2 tbsp Mayo
- 1 tbsp Dijon mustard
- 1 tsp of fresh lime juice
- Salt & pepper

Additional ingredients:

- 1 sliced tomato
- 1 sliced avocado
- 2 sliced hard boiled eggs

INSTRUCTIONS

1. Microwave your cauliflower for 4-5 minutes and drain very well using a cheesecloth or towel. Combine all ingredients for the cauliflower portion of the recipe and mix well.

2. combine and mix all ingredients for the tuna salad portion.

3. Line plastic wrap to a small deep bowl/dish

4. Layer cauliflower, tuna and make sure to pack it in well.

5. Add a layer of tomatoes, hard boiled eggs, and avocado.

6. Add final layer of cauliflower and flip into a flat dish, remove plastic wrap

7. Add a thin layer of Mayo and garnish

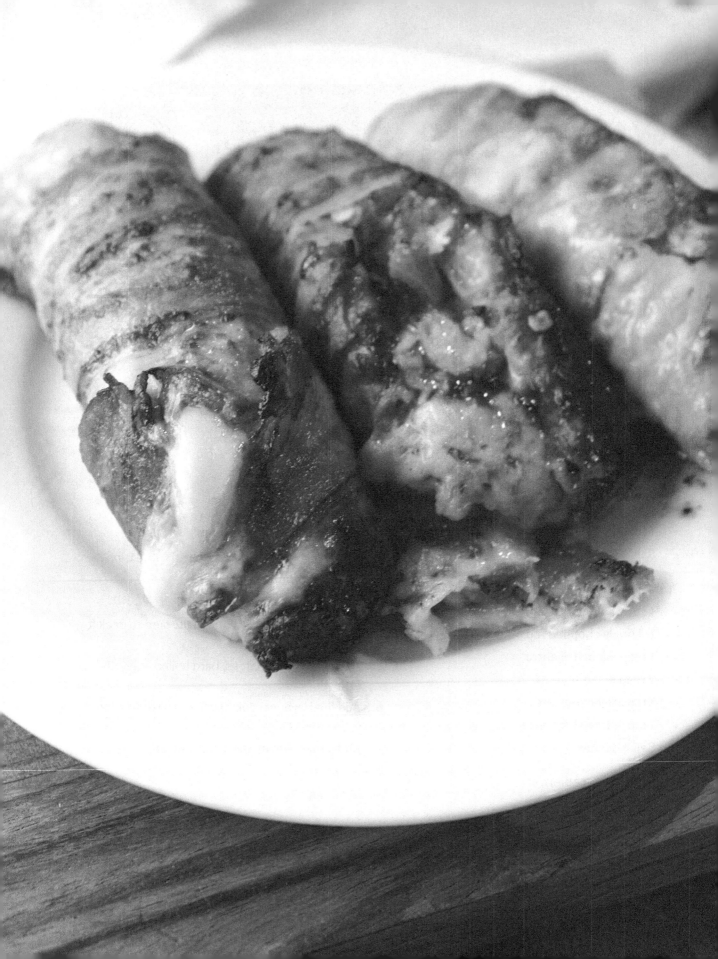

Cheddar Stuffed Bacon Wrapped Brats

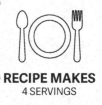

RECIPE MAKES
4 SERVINGS

MACROS

💧 **CAL: 397G** 🛢 **FAT: 34G** 🍳 **PROTEIN: 21G**

🌾 **TOTAL CARBS: 1G** 🌿 **FIBER: 0G** 🌾 **NET CARBS: 1G**

INGREDIENTS

- 5 bratwursts
- 5 sticks of cheddar
- 5 slices of bacon

Optional:

- Onions & Jalapeños

INSTRUCTIONS

1. Cut a slit into your bratwursts & stuff with the cheddar sticks.

2. Wrap with bacon.

3. Air fry at 400F for 10-15 minutes.

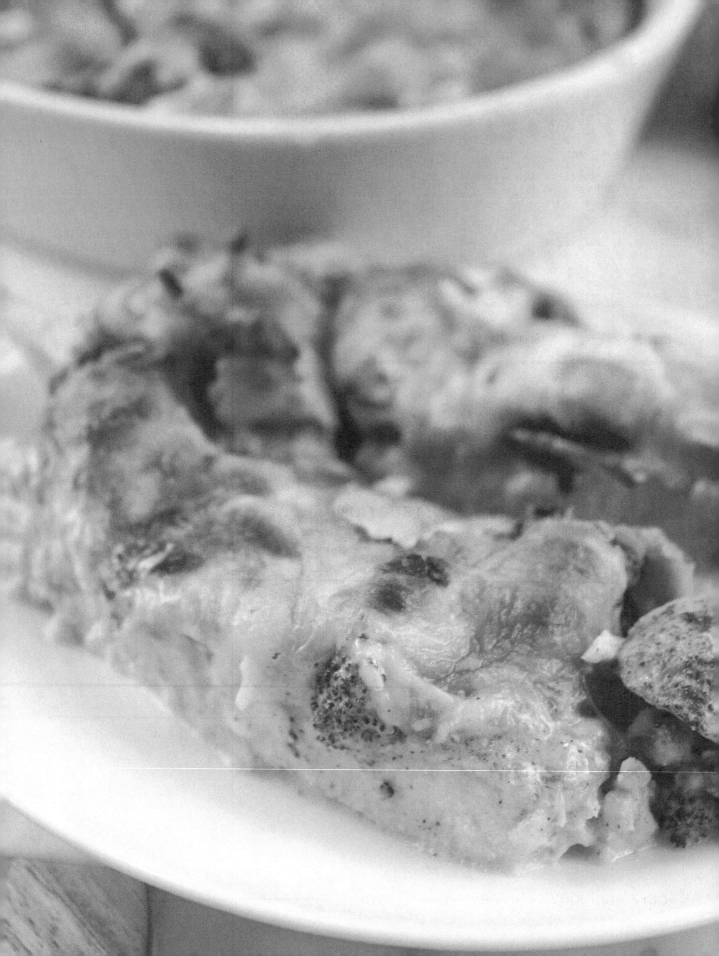

Chicken Bacon Ranch Casserole

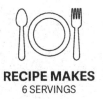

RECIPE MAKES
6 SERVINGS

MACROS

🔥 CAL: 428   🛢 FAT: 35G   🥚 PROTEIN: 24G

🌾 TOTAL CARBS: 6G   🍃 FIBER: 1G   🌾 NET CARBS: 5G

INGREDIENTS

- 4 thinly sliced chicken breasts
- 2 tbsp butter
- 2 cups fresh broccoli, chopped
- 1/2 cup ranch dressing
- 3/4 cup shredded mozzarella
- 2 cups shredded cheddar
- 3 slices bacon, chopped
- 1 tsp garlic powder
- 1 tsp paprika
- Salt & pepper

INSTRUCTIONS

1. Preheat oven to 375F.
2. Melt butter & add to the bottom of a 9x13 baking dish.
3. Season your chicken and add to baking dish.
4. Add broccoli, bacon, ranch, mozzarella, & top with cheddar.
5. Bake for 30 minutes. Take out, let cool, & enjoy!

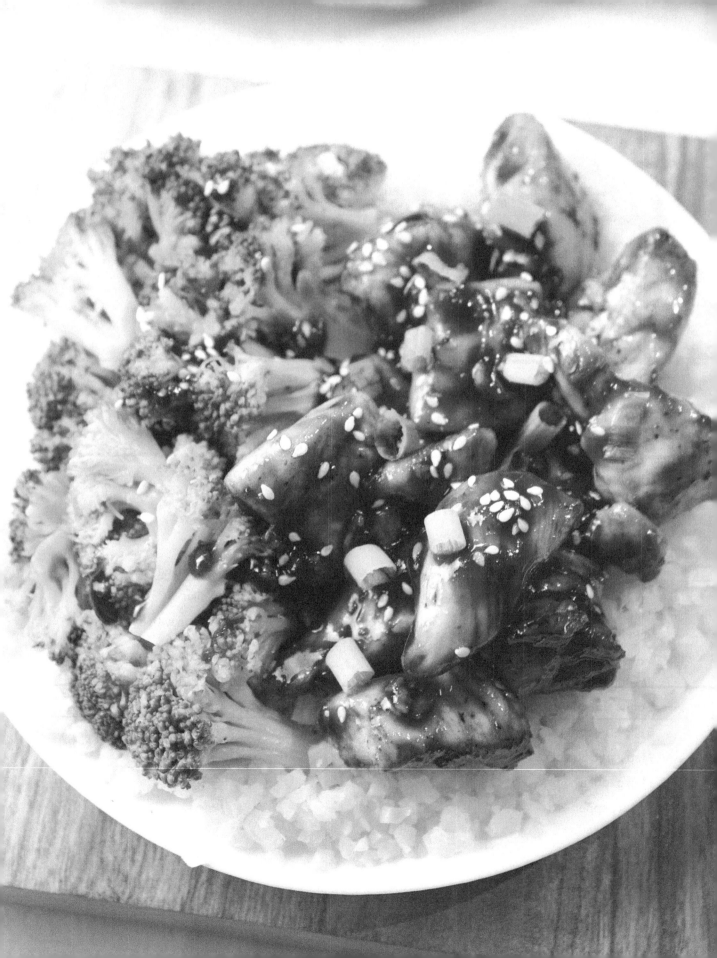

Chicken Teriyaki

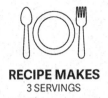

RECIPE MAKES
3 SERVINGS

MACROS

🔥 **CAL: 418**   💧 **FAT: 23G**   🍖 **PROTEIN: 49G**

🌾 **TOTAL CARBS: 3G**   🌿 **FIBER: 0.3G**   🌾 **NET CARBS: 2.7G**

INGREDIENTS

- 1.5 lb chicken thighs
- 2 tbsp avocado oil
- 1 tsp sesame seeds
- Salt & pepper

For the Sauce:

- 1/2 cup soy sauce
- 1 tbsp avocado oil
- 3/4 cup water
- 1 tbsp red wine vinegar
- 1 tsp ground ginger
- 1 tsp garlic powder
- 3 tbsp sweetener
- 1/4 teaspoon xanthan gum

INSTRUCTIONS

1. Mix all ingredients for the sauce and add to a saucepan over medium heat

2. Let cook for 5-10 minutes. Remove from heat and set aside.

3. Chop your chicken thighs into bite sized pieces and season with salt & pepper.

4. Add to a large skillet with oil over medium high heat and cook for 4-5 minutes. (Until internal temp reaches 165F)

5. Remove from heat, mix with sauce, & serve with your favorite side!

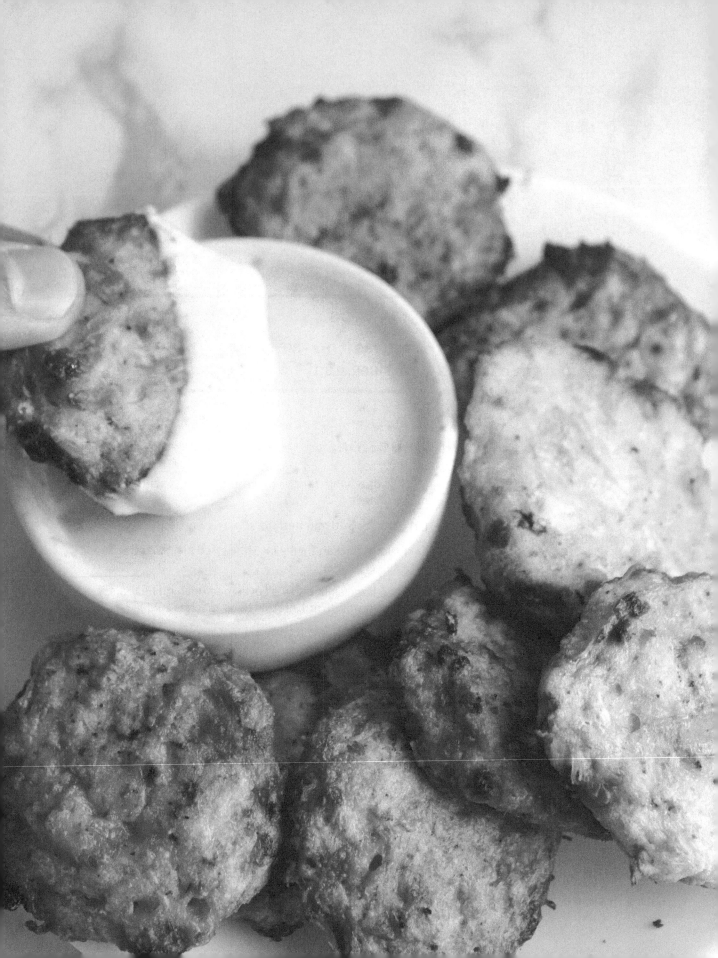

Chicken Nuggets

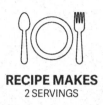

RECIPE MAKES
2 SERVINGS

MACROS

 CAL: 260   **FAT: 12G**   **PROTEIN: 34G**

 TOTAL CARBS: 1G   **FIBER: 0G**   **NET CARBS: 1G**

INGREDIENTS

- 12 oz fully cooked chunk chicken breast, drained
- 1 large egg
- 1/2 cup shredded cheddar cheese
- Seasonings of your choice

INSTRUCTIONS

1. Combine all ingredients and shape into nuggets.
2. Bake at 400F for 20 minutes.
3. Take out, let cool, & enjoy!

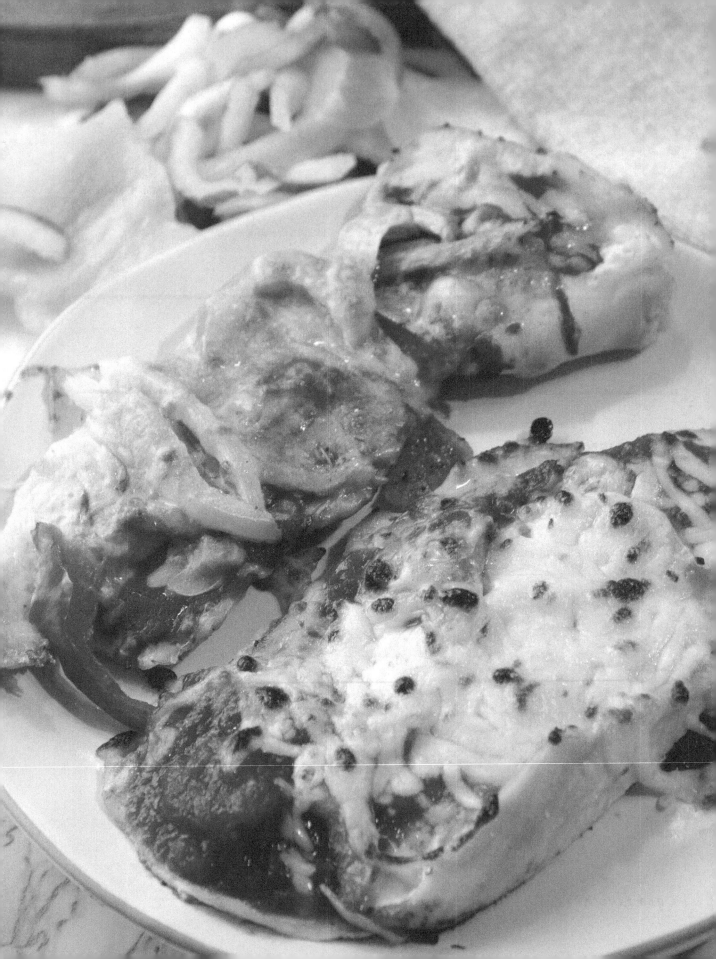

Chicken Cutlet Pizza

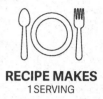

RECIPE MAKES
1 SERVING

MACROS (For traditional style only)

🔥 **CAL:** 453   🔥 **FAT:** 18G   🍳 **PROTEIN:** 67G

🌾 **TOTAL CARBS:** 6G   🌿 **FIBER:** 0.1G   🌾 **NET CARBS:** 5.9G

INGREDIENTS

- 4 sliced chicken breasts (extra thin)

Traditional:

- ½ cup shredded mozzarella
- ¼ cup marinara sauce
- ¼ cup peppers and onions
- 1 tsp oregano
- 1/2 tsp dried oregano
- Salt & pepper

Mexican style:

- ¼ cup queso / cheese sauce
- ½ cup shredded cheddar
- ¼ cup peppers & onions
- 1 tsp cumin
- ½ tsp chili powder
- Salt & pepper

INSTRUCTIONS

1. Season your chicken & bake at 400F for 15 minutes, until internal temp reaches 165F.

2. Take out, add your toppings & broil until the cheese melts.

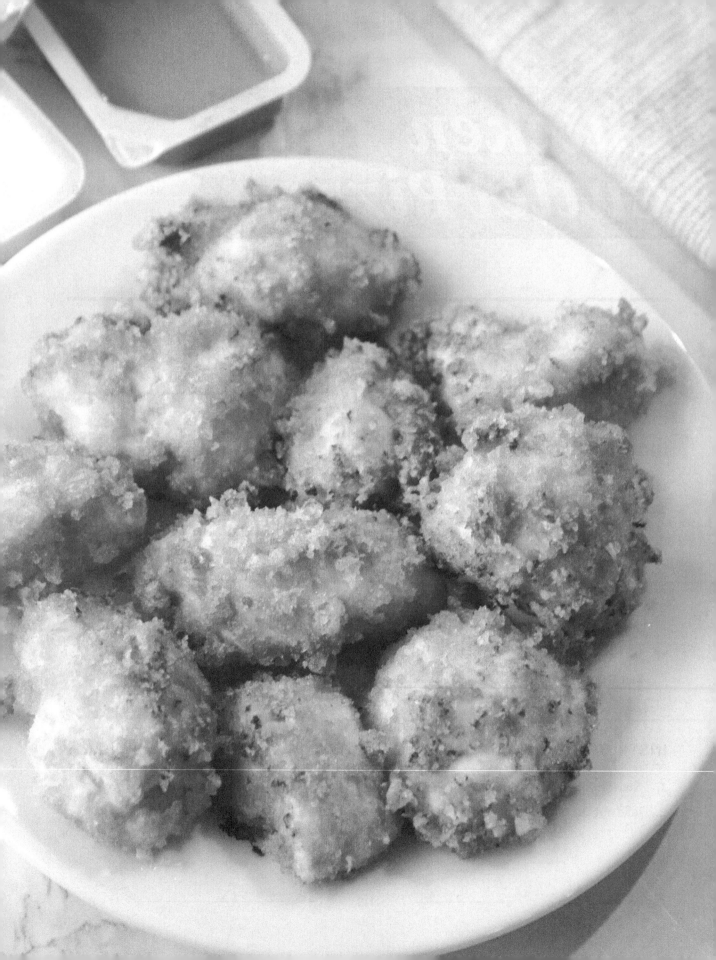

Chick Fil A Nuggets

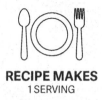

RECIPE MAKES
1 SERVING

MACROS (For 1/2 recipe)

🔥 **CAL: 577**   🛢 **FAT: 25G**   🍳 **PROTEIN: 90G**

🌾 **TOTAL CARBS: 0G**   🍃 **FIBER: 9G**   🌾 **NET CARBS: 3G**

INGREDIENTS

- 1 cup pickle juice
- 1 lb boneless skinless chicken breast
- 1 large egg
- 4 oz pork rinds

INSTRUCTIONS

1. Cut your chicken into nugget sized pieces and marinate in the pickle juice for 30 minutes. (The longer the better)

2. Blend your pork rinds, whisk your egg & drain the pickle juice from the chicken.

3. Coat your chicken in the egg and then in the pork rind crumbs.

4. Air fry for 10 minutes at 400F & enjoy!

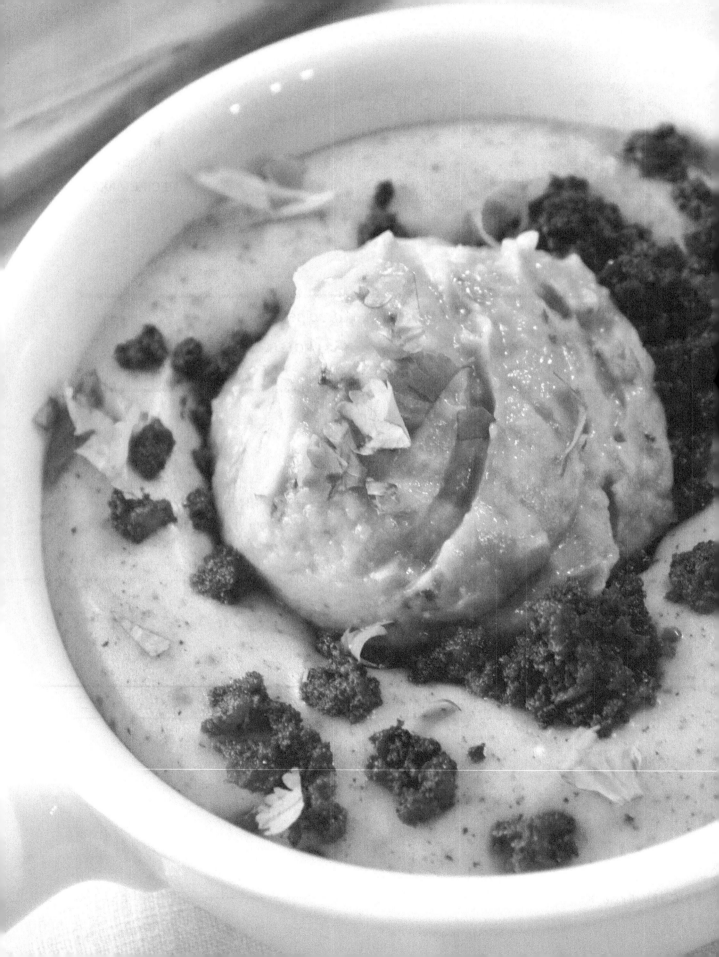

Chori Queso Dip

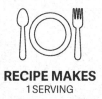

RECIPE MAKES
1 SERVING

MACROS (For 1/4 recipe)

🔥 CAL: 430   🫗 FAT: 36G   🍳 PROTEIN: 22G

🌾 TOTAL CARBS: 4G   🍃 FIBER: 0G   🌾 NET CARBS: 4G

INGREDIENTS

- 8 oz chorizo
- 1/2 cup heavy cream
- 2 cups shredded Mexican blend cheese

Optional:

- Guacamole
- Cilantro

INSTRUCTIONS

1. In a skillet cook the chorizo, add to a strainer to drain the grease, pat dry & set aside.

2. In the same skillet add your heavy cream & shredded cheese.

3. Stir for 3-5 minutes.

4. Remove from heat, add your chorizo, guacamole, & cilantro.

5. Serve warm, dip with your favorite keto friendly chips or veggies & enjoy!

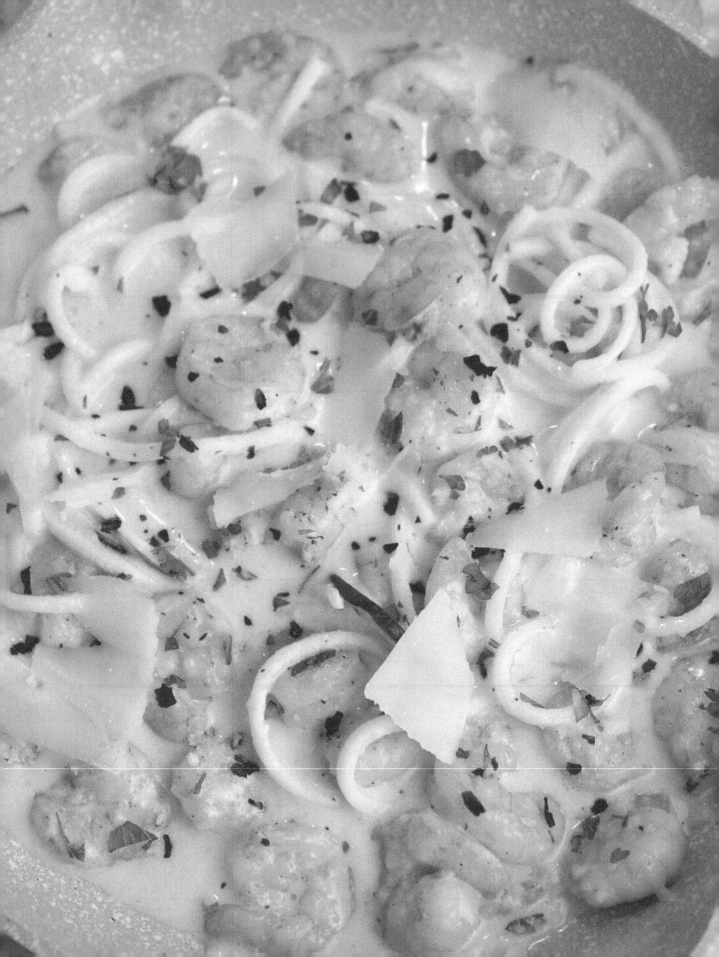

Creamy Garlic Shrimp

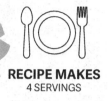

RECIPE MAKES
4 SERVINGS

MACROS

🔥 **CAL: 415**   🫗 **FAT: 29G**   🥚 **PROTEIN: 29G**

🌾 **TOTAL CARBS: 4G**   🍃 **FIBER: 0G**   🌾 **NET CARBS: 4G**

INGREDIENTS

- 3 tbsp avocado oil
- 1 lb fresh shrimp (10)
- 2 tbsp butter
- 1 tbsp minced garlic
- 1/4 cup white wine (Chardonay)
- 1/2 cup heavy cream
- 1/2 cup grated parmesan
- Salt & pepper

INSTRUCTIONS

1. Season the shrimp and add to skillet with oil on medium heat.

2. Cook for 2 minutes on each side. Remove from pan and set aside.

3. Add butter to pan on medium low and add your garlic until fragrant.

4. Add the wine and let it reduce.

5. Add the heavy cream and parmesan and let it continue to reduce.

6. Finish by adding salt, parsley, and your shrimp.

7. Remove from heat & enjoy!

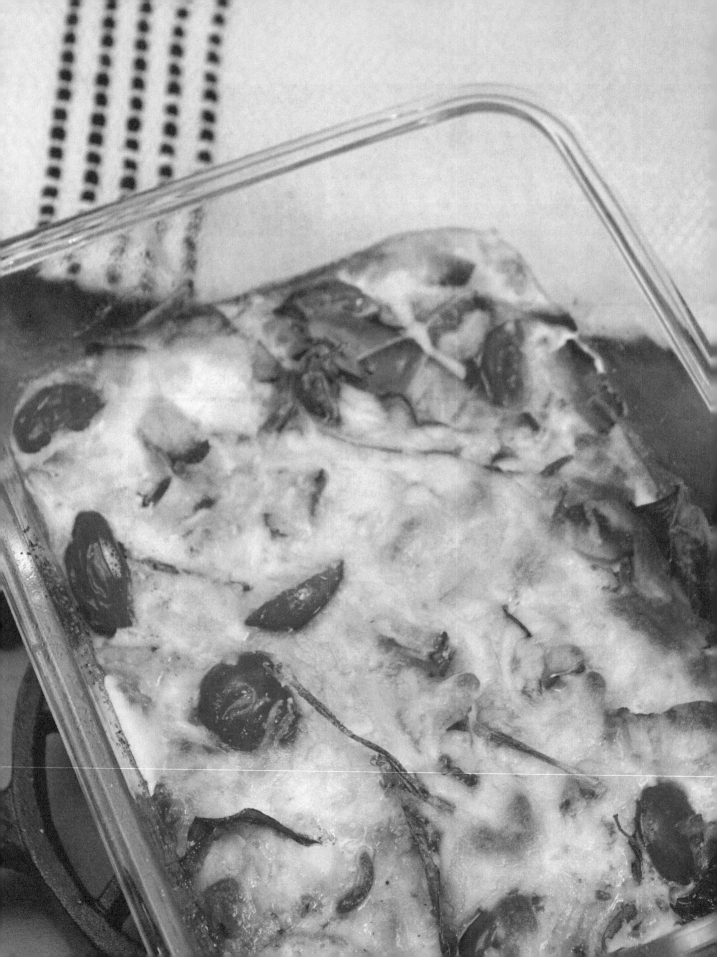

Egg Frittata

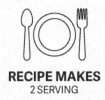

RECIPE MAKES
2 SERVING

MACROS

🔥 **CAL: 358**   🥑 **FAT: 30G**   🥚 **PROTEIN: 21G**

🌾 **TOTAL CARBS: 4G**   🍃 **FIBER: 2G**   🌾 **NET CARBS: 2G**

INGREDIENTS

- 6 large eggs
- 1/2 cup fresh spinach
- 1/4 cup chopped ham
- 1/4 cup chopped tomatoes
- 1/2 cup shredded Mexican cheese

INSTRUCTIONS

1.   Line a baking dish with parchment paper & spray with oil.

2.   Add your eggs & top with remaining ingredients.

3.   Sprinkle salt, pepper & your favorite seasonings on top.

4.   Bake at 350F for 25 minutes, take out when it's no longer jiggly in the middle & enjoy!

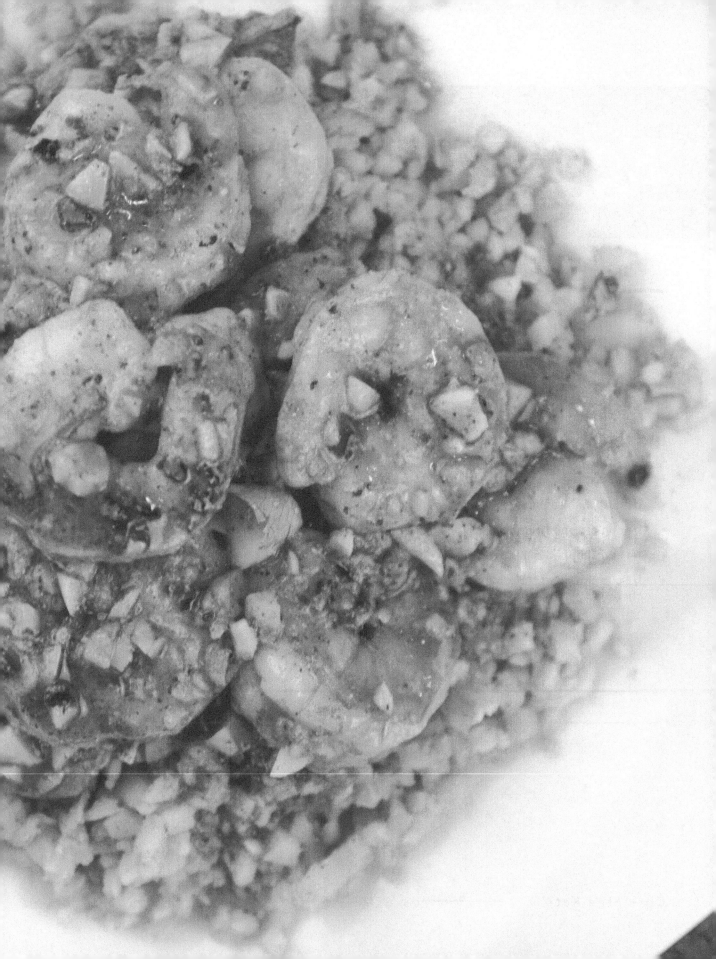

Garlic Parmesan Shrimp & Cauliflower Rice

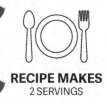

RECIPE MAKES
2 SERVINGS

MACROS

🔥 **CAL: 662**   🫗 **FAT: 27G**   🥚 **PROTEIN: 75G**

🌾 **TOTAL CARBS: 11.5G**   🍃 **FIBER: 3G**   🌾 **NET CARBS: 8.5G**

INGREDIENTS

- 1.5 lbs raw shrimp, peeled and deveined
- 1 head cauliflower florets, riced
- 1/4 cup butter
- 1/3 cup chicken broth
- 1/2 onion, chopped
- 4 cloves garlic, minced
- 1 tsp Italian seasoning
- 2 tsp onion powder
- 1.5 tbsp sriracha
- 3 oz fresh grated parmesan
- 1 oz lemon juice
- 1 tsp red pepper flakes
- Fresh parsley, chopped
- Salt & pepper

INSTRUCTIONS

1. Season shrimp with salt & pepper. Set aside.
2. Heat a large skillet over medium heat with 2 tbsp butter. Add 2 cloves of minced garlic, & your chopped onion for 1 minute. (Until fragrant)
3. Add the riced cauliflower to the pan and stir until everything is coated with butter.
4. Stir in 2 tbsp chicken broth & 1 tbsp parsley. Cook for 1 minute and then add 2 oz parmesan.
5. Cook for 1 more minute, remove from pan, & set aside.
6. In the same pan melt 2 tbsp butter and add your seasoned shrimp, minced garlic, Italian seasoning, & onion powder.
7. Stir to combine & cook shrimp for 1-2 minutes on each side.
8. Add your remaining chicken broth, sriracha, & parmesan and cook for 1 more minute.
9. Lower heat to simmer and add your riced cauliflower. Mix together to reheat & remove from heat.
10. Top with lemon juice, red pepper flakes and parsley. Serve & enjoy!

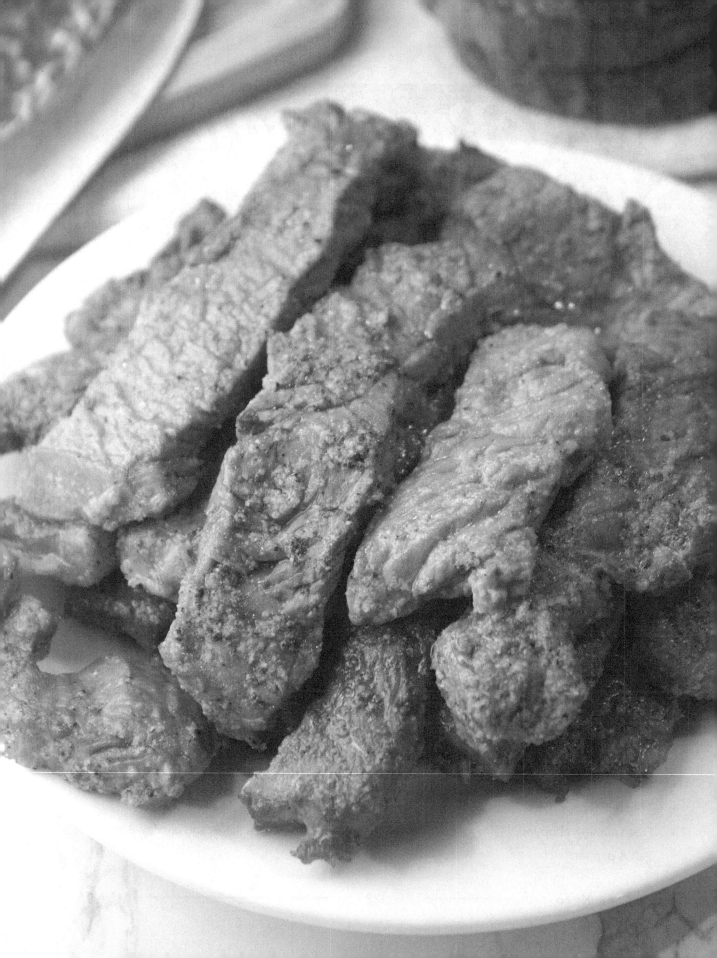

Garlic Butter Steak Bites

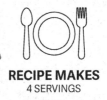

RECIPE MAKES
4 SERVINGS

MACROS

🔥 CAL: 539   🟠 FAT: 28G   🍳 PROTEIN: 67G

🌾 TOTAL CARBS: 0G   🍃 FIBER: 0G   🌾 NET CARBS: 0G

INGREDIENTS

- 2 lbs steak
- 4 tbsp butter, melted
- 2 tsp garlic powder
- Salt & pepper

INSTRUCTIONS

1. Season your steak with salt & pepper. Let rest at room temp for 30 minutes.

2. Melt your butter in a large mixing bowl.

3. Add the steak & garlic to your bowl and mix.

4. Air fry at 400F for 5-6 minutes.

5. Take out, let cool, & enjoy!

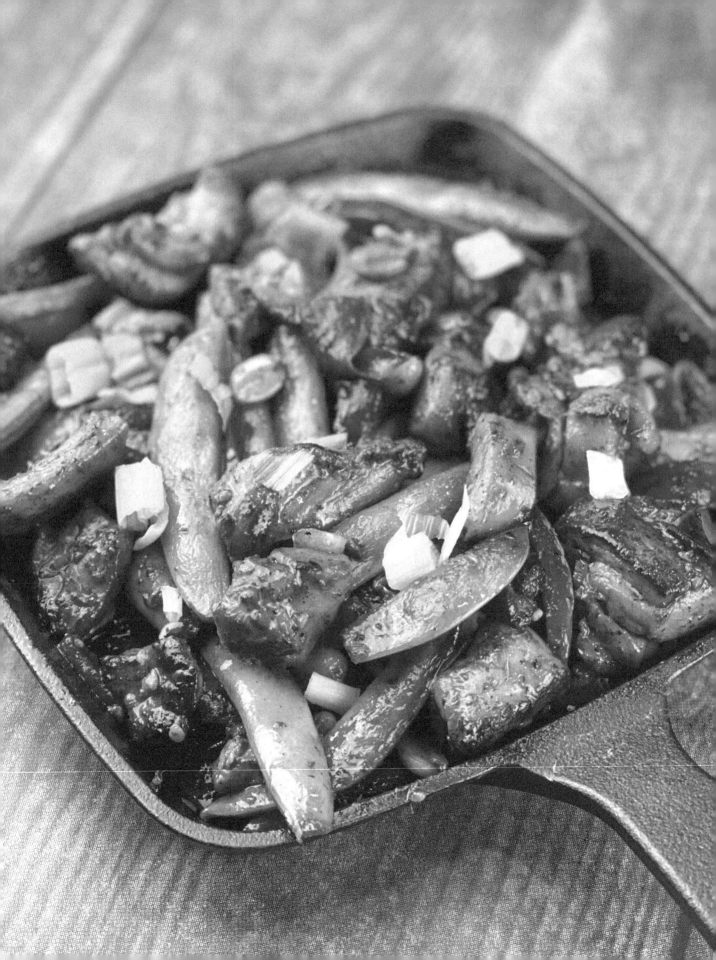

Kung Pao Chicken

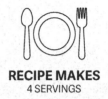

RECIPE MAKES
4 SERVINGS

MACROS

🔥 CAL: 252   🫗 FAT: 15G   🥄 PROTEIN: 21.5G

🌾 TOTAL CARBS: 7.5G   🌿 FIBER: 3G   🌾 NET CARBS: 4.5G

INGREDIENTS

Chicken

- 1 lb chicken thigh or breast cut into cubes
- 1 tsp soy sauce
- 1 tsp sherry
- 1/2 tsp sweetener
- 1/2 tsp starch (or psyllium husk)
- Salt & pepper to taste

Stir fry sauce

- 1/4 cup chicken broth
- 2 tsp starch (or psyllium husk)
- 1 tbsp soy sauce
- 1 tbsp sweetener
- 1 tbsp sherry
- 1 tbsp white vinegar

Stir fry

- 2 tbsp avocado oil
- 1 red bell pepper
- 2 cups sugar snap peas
- 2 cloves minced garlic
- 2 tsp fresh ginger
- Peanuts (optional)
- Green onion (optional)

INSTRUCTIONS

1. Mix chicken with ingredients and let sit for 15 mins.

2. Cook the chicken on medium high with 1 tbsp oil and set aside.

3. Whisk together stir fry sauce, set aside.

4. In 2 tbsp oil cook peppers & sugar snap peas for 2-3 mins until tender.

5. Stir in garlic and ginger and cook for 30 seconds.

6. Add chicken back to pan & toss together.

7. Stir in the sauce to combine all ingredients. Add peanuts.

8. Let simmer until it thickens.

9. Top with green onion & peanuts!

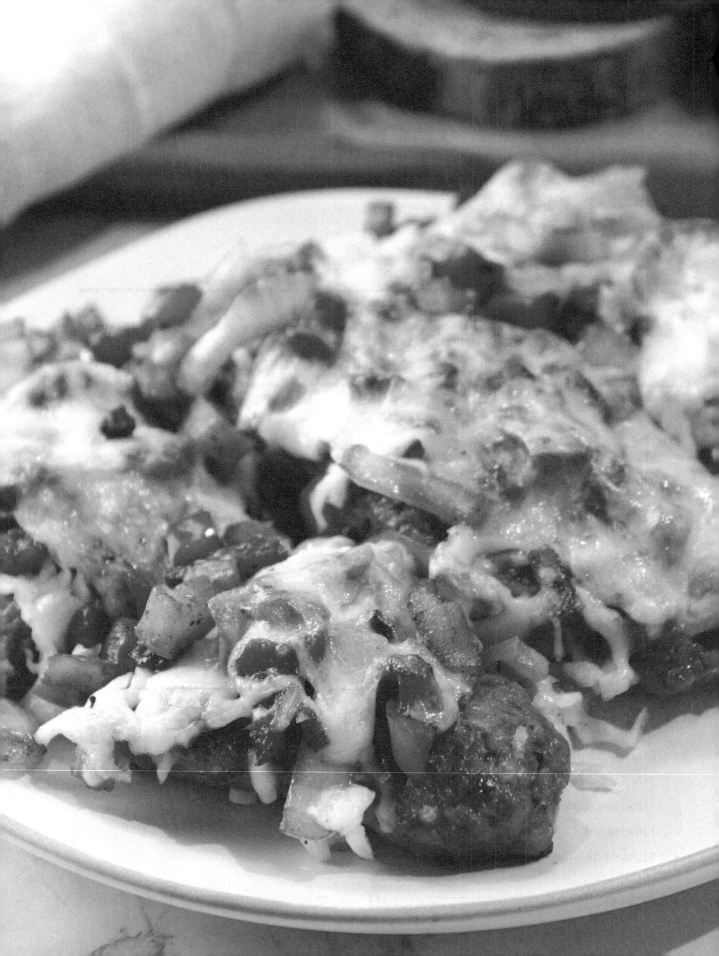

Loaded Sausages

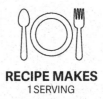

RECIPE MAKES
1 SERVING

MACROS (For 1/4 recipe)

🔥 **CAL: 320**   🥑 **FAT: 23G**   🍲 **PROTEIN: 24G**

🌾 **TOTAL CARBS: 5G**   🍃 **FIBER: 0.2G**   🌾 **NET CARBS: 4.8G**

INGREDIENTS

- 4 Italian sausage links
- 3/4 cup sliced peppers & onions
- 2 slices of provolone
- 1/2 cup shredded mozzarella
- 1/4 cup balsamic vinegar

INSTRUCTIONS

1. Cut your sausage in half and flatten.

2. Pan fry both sides on medium heat until fully cooked. Remove from pan but leave in the grease.

3. Add your onions & peppers to the pan with the balsamic vinegar.

4. Once caramelized remove from heat and set aside.

5. Add your sausage to a baking dish & top with the pepper mix, provolone, & mozzarella.

6. Broil until cheese melts & enjoy!

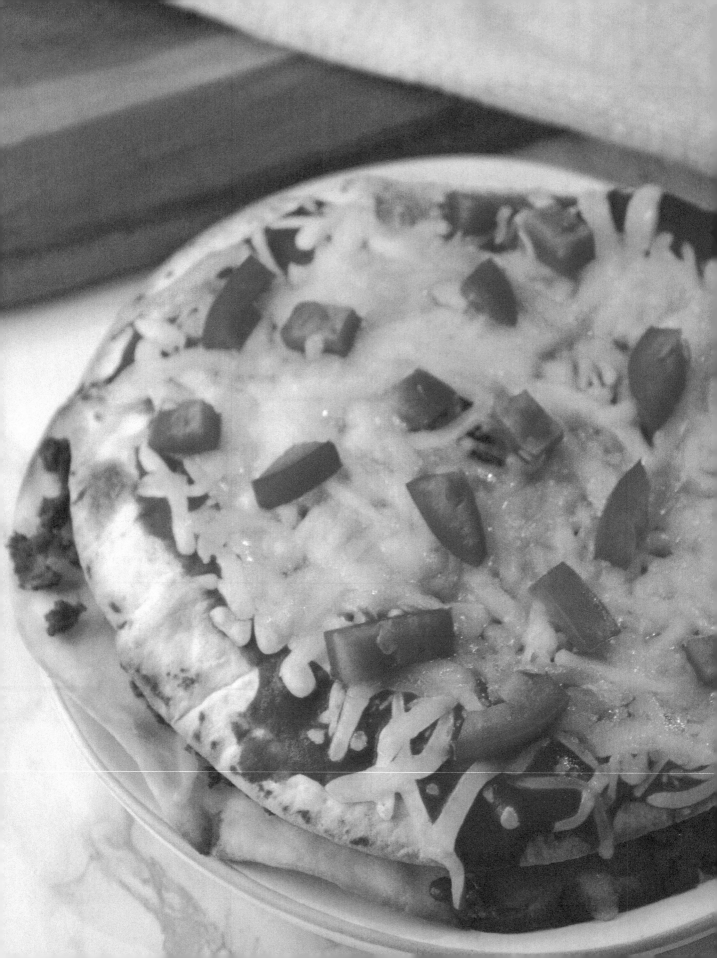

Mexican Pizza

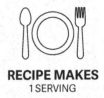

RECIPE MAKES
1 SERVING

MACROS (For 1/2 pizza)

🔥 CAL: 298   🫗 FAT: 16G   🫘 PROTEIN: 21G

🌾 TOTAL CARBS: 16G   🌿 FIBER: 10G   🌾 NET CARBS: 6G

INGREDIENTS

- 2 low carb tortillas
- 4 oz beef, cooked w/ taco seasoning
- 1/4 cup Mexican blend cheese
- 2 tomato slices
- 1/4 cup red enchilada sauce
- 3 tbsp avocado oil

INSTRUCTIONS

1. Add avocado oil to a pan over medium heat.
2. Add the tortillas and cook on both sides until crispy.
3. Remove from pan and pat dry with paper towels.
4. Top one tortilla with ground beef and the other tortilla.
5. Spread the sauce on top of that along with your tomatoes and cheese.
6. Broil until the cheese melts.
7. Enjoy!

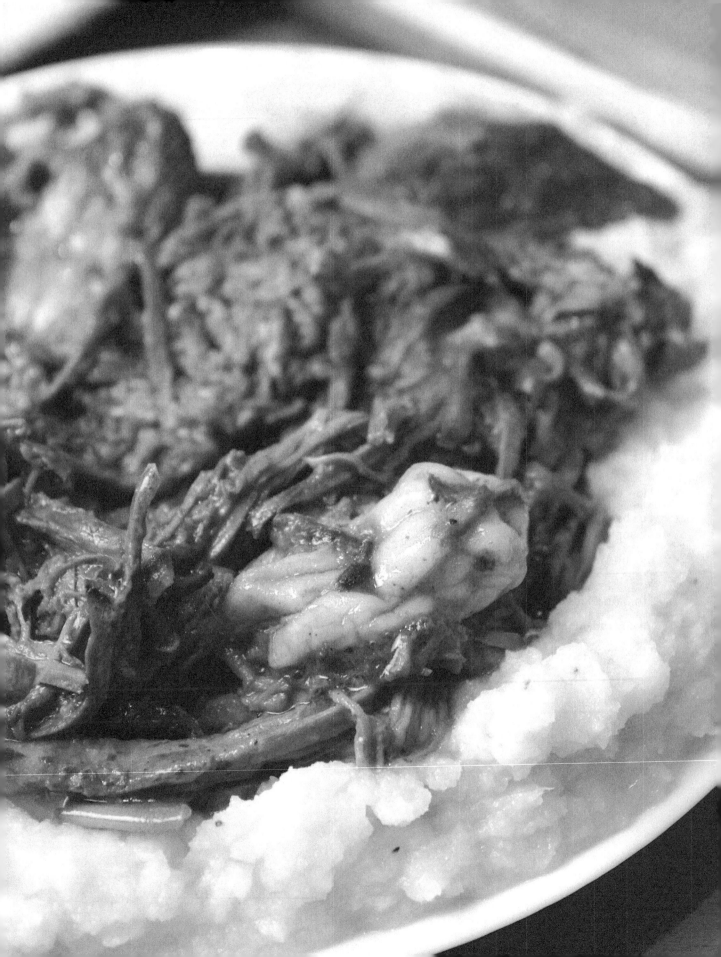

Mississippi Pot Roast

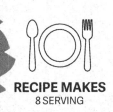

RECIPE MAKES
8 SERVING

MACROS

🔥 CAL: 427   🛢 FAT: 21G   🥚 PROTEIN: 56G

🌾 TOTAL CARBS: 1G   🍃 FIBER: 0G   🌾 NET CARBS: 1G

INGREDIENTS

- 3 lb chuck roast
- 1 packet of ranch seasoning
- 1 packet of AU Jus Gravy seasoning
- 1/2 stick of butter
- 5-6 pepperoncini

INSTRUCTIONS

1. Brown your roast on all sides & add to the slow cooker with the rest of your ingredients.

2. Cook on low for 8 hours.

3. Serve over mashed cauliflower & enjoy!!

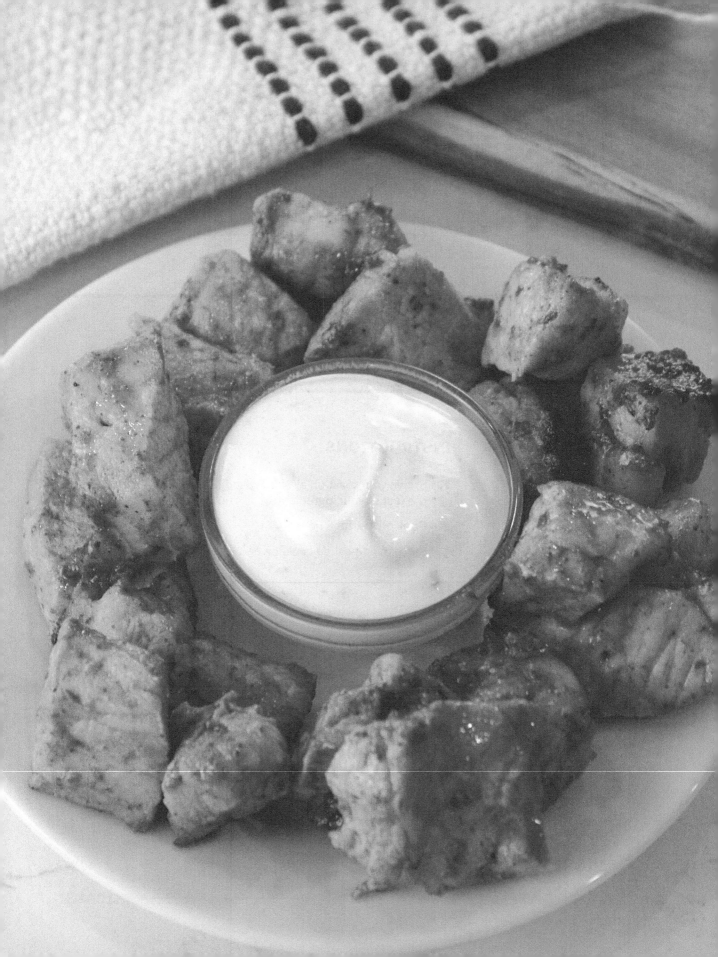

Pork Chop Ranch Bites

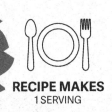

RECIPE MAKES
1 SERVING

MACROS (For 1/4 recipe)

CAL: 268   FAT: 17G   PROTEIN: 24G
TOTAL CARBS: 3G   FIBER: 9G   NET CARBS: 3G

INGREDIENTS

- 1 lb pork chops
- 3 tbsp avocado oil
- 4 tbsp ranch seasoning

INSTRUCTIONS

1. Cut your pork chops into bite sized pieces.

2. Mix in a large bowl with oil & seasoning.

3. Air fry at 400F for 10 minutes.

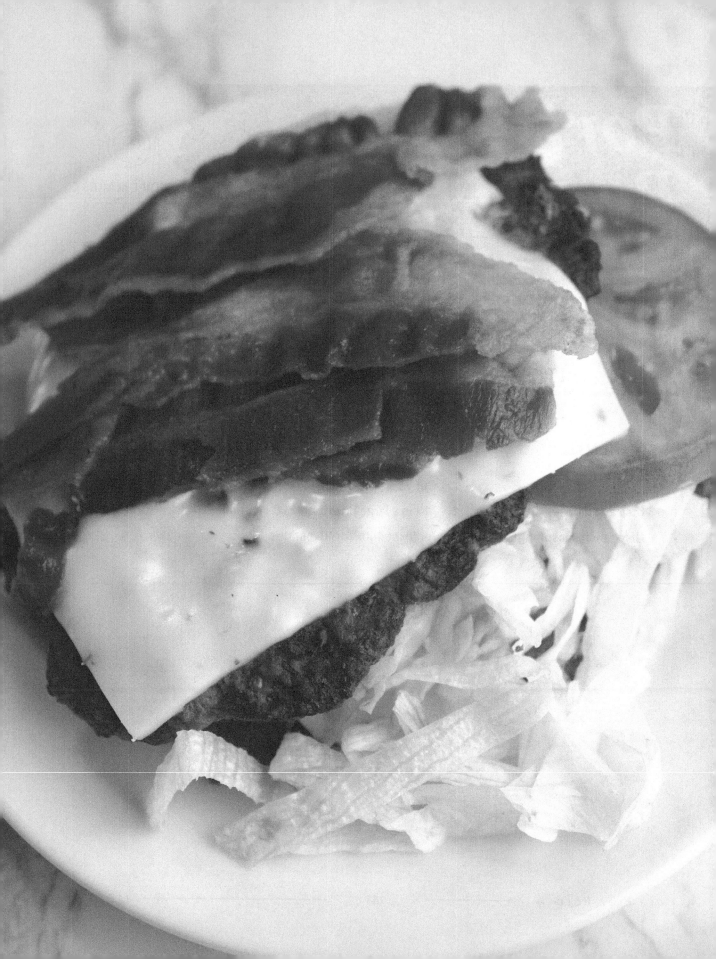

Pepper Jack Burger

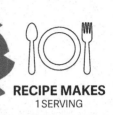

RECIPE MAKES
1 SERVING

MACROS

🔥 CAL: 736   🫗 FAT: 52G   🥚 PROTEIN: 60G

🌾 TOTAL CARBS: 3G   🍃 FIBER: 0.3G   🌾 NET CARBS: 27G

INGREDIENTS

- 8 oz ground beef
- 2 slices pepper Jack cheese
- 2 slices bacon, fully cooked
- 1/2 cup shredded lettuce
- 1 tomato slice
- Salt & pepper

INSTRUCTIONS

1. Mix your beef with salt & pepper.

2. Shape into 2 patties and fry on medium high for 2 minutes on each side.

3. Add your cheese on top for the last minute and cover until it melts.

4. Combine with the rest of your ingredients & enjoy!

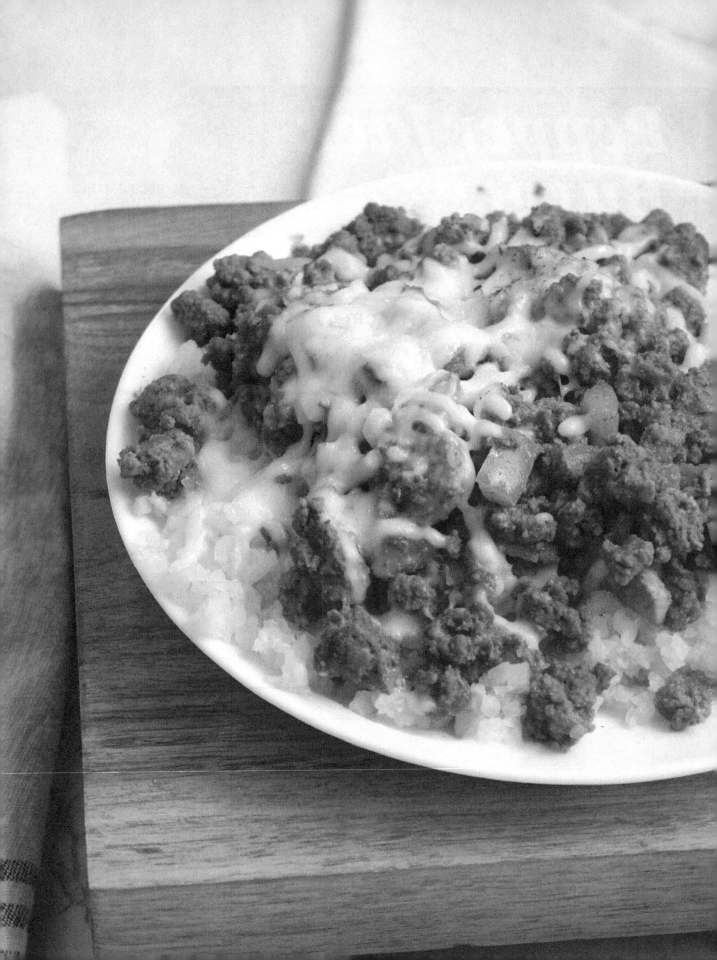

Philly Cheesesteak Skillet

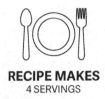

RECIPE MAKES
4 SERVINGS

MACROS

🔥 **CAL: 513**　　💧 **FAT: 28G**　　🍳 **PROTEIN: 51G**

🌾 **TOTAL CARBS: 13.5G**　　🍃 **FIBER: 3.3G**　　🌾 **NET CARBS: 10.2G**

INGREDIENTS

- 1.5 lbs beef
- 6 oz provolone cheese
- 8 oz fresh cauliflower rice, drained
- 2 tbsp oil
- 1 yellow onion, thinly sliced
- 1 green bell pepper, thinly sliced
- 8 oz mushrooms, thinly sliced
- 2 cloves garlic, minced
- 1 tbsp Dijon mustard
- 2 tbsp coconut aminos
- Salt & pepper

INSTRUCTIONS

I. In a skillet over medium heat add the olive oil, cauliflower rice, onion, & peppers stirring occasionally for 5-7 minutes. Once browned remove from pan & set aside.

2. In the pan add your minced garlic until fragrant and then add the beef, salt & pepper. Cook until browned and drain the fat.

3. Add the beef back to your pan along with everything else except the provolone. Cook for 2-3 minutes until bubbly.

4. Place your cheese on top and cover until it melts or simply place under the broiler for 1-2 minutes.

5. Take out, let cool, & enjoy!

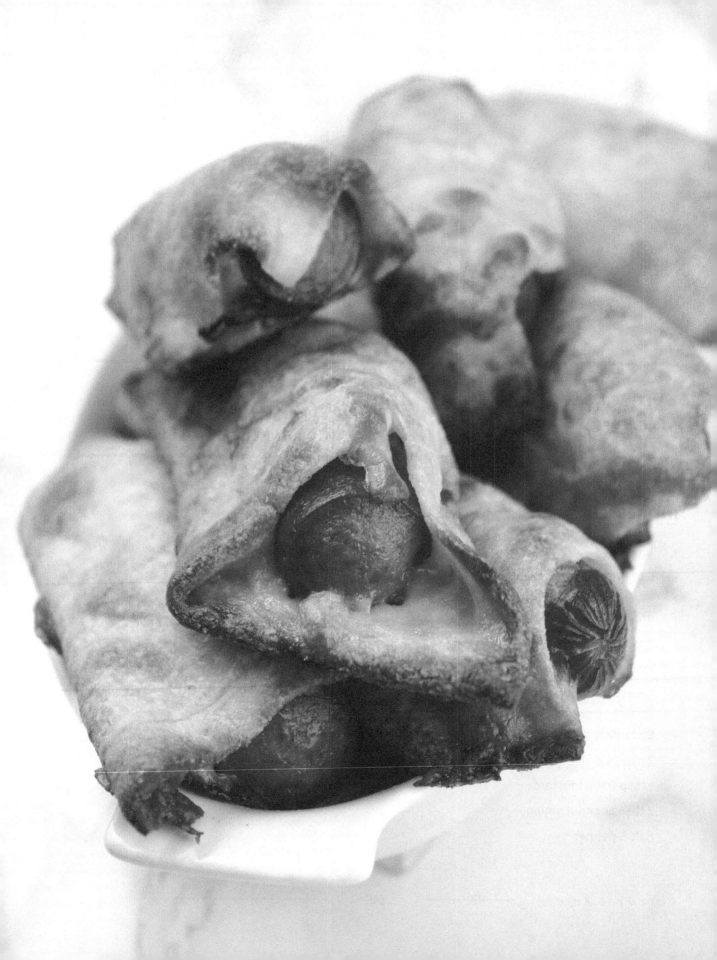

Pigs in a Blanket

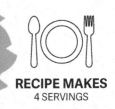

RECIPE MAKES
4 SERVINGS

MACROS

🔥 **CAL:** 546   🫗 **FAT:** 48G   🥄 **PROTEIN:** 23G

🌾 **TOTAL CARBS:** 8G   🍃 **FIBER:** 3G   🌾 **NET CARBS:** 5G

INGREDIENTS

- 8 hot dogs (halved)
- 1 1/2 cup shredded mozzarella
- 2 tbsp cream cheese
- 1 cup almond flour
- 1 large egg (whisked)
- salt & pepper

INSTRUCTIONS

1. Preheat the oven to 350F.

2. Mix cream cheese and mozzarella. Microwave for 1 minute. Stir and microwave for 30 more seconds. Stir again.

3. Add your whisked egg & almond flour. Mix.

4. Add your seasonings and mix again.

5. Knead and flatten out between two sheets of greased parchment paper.

6. Cut into 2x2 inch rectangles, add your hot dogs and roll them up.

7. Bake for 20 minutes until the dough is golden brown.

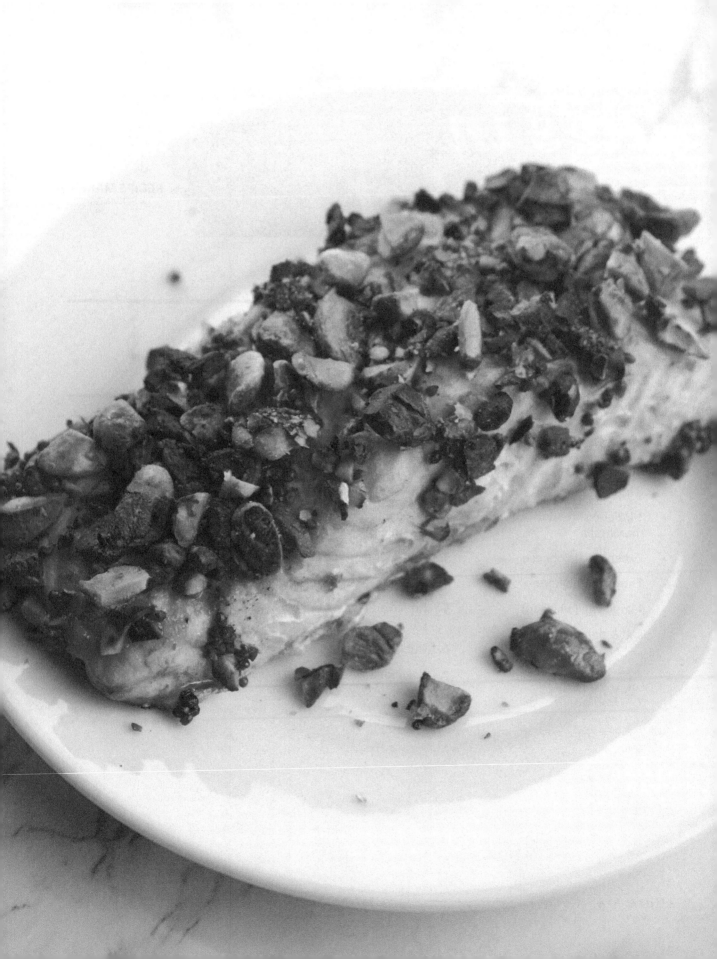

Pistachio Crusted Salmon

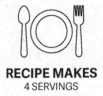

RECIPE MAKES
4 SERVINGS

MACROS

🔥 **CAL: 250**   💧 **FAT: 11G**   🍳 **PROTEIN: 27G**

🌾 **TOTAL CARBS: 10G**   🐟 **FIBER: 2.5G**   🌾 **NET CARBS: 7.5G**

INGREDIENTS

- 16 oz salmon
- 1/3 cup pistachios
- 3 tbsp ground Dijon mustard
- 1-2 tbsp sugar free maple syrup
- Salt & pepper

INSTRUCTIONS

1. Preheat oven to 400F & line a baking sheet with foil.
2. Chop up your pistachios & set aside.
3. Combine Dijon with syrup, salt, & pepper.
4. Spread the Dijon mix on your salmon, press the salmon down into the chopped pistachios and coat all sides.
5. Bake for 12 minutes. Let cool, & enjoy!

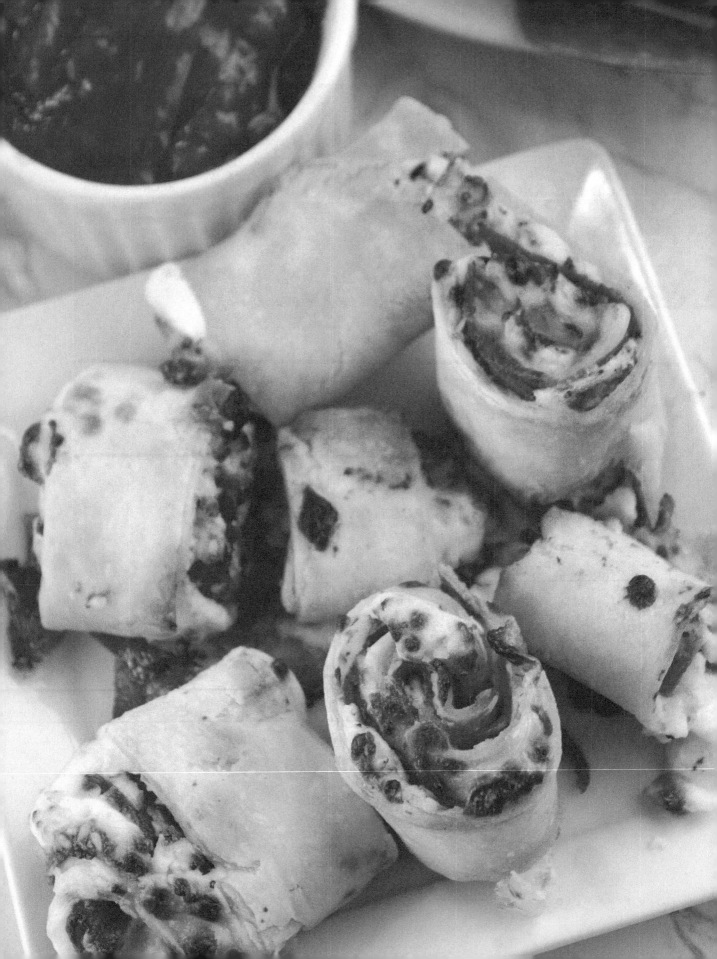

Pizza Pinwheels

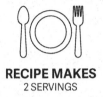

RECIPE MAKES
2 SERVINGS

MACROS

🔥 **CAL: 624**   🫗 **FAT: 30G**   🥩 **PROTEIN: 7G**

🌾 **TOTAL CARBS: 7G**   🍃 **FIBER: 5G**   🌾 **NET CARBS: 2G**

INGREDIENTS

- 1 low carb tortilla
- 3 oz butter
- 2 oz cream cheese, room temp
- 1/4 cup shredded mozzarella
- 8 pepperoni slices
- 1 tsp everything bagel seasoning

INSTRUCTIONS

1. Melt your butter and coat one side of your tortilla.
2. On the other side, spread your cream cheese & add the rest of your ingredients.
3. Roll up tightly, slice into 6-8 pieces.
4. Air fry at 400F for 6-8 minutes. (Until golden brown & crispy)

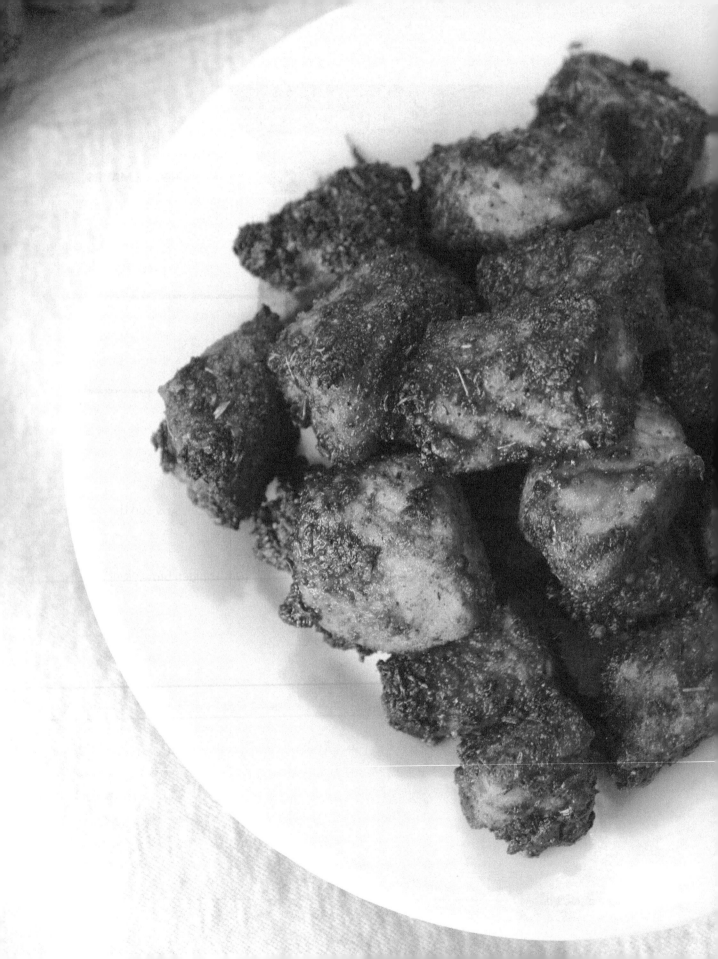

Pork Chop Bites

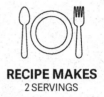

RECIPE MAKES
2 SERVINGS

MACROS

🔥 **CAL: 530**   💧 **FAT: 34G**   🥚 **PROTEIN: 49G**

🌾 **TOTAL CARBS: 1.5G**   🍃 **FIBER: 0G**   🌾 **NET CARBS: 1.5G**

INGREDIENTS

- 1 lb pork chops
- 3 tbsp oil
- 1 tsp paprika
- 1 tsp chili powder
- 1/2 tsp garlic powder
- 1/2 tsp onion powder
- 1/2 tsp dried thyme
- 1/4 tsp cayenne pepper
- Salt & black pepper

INSTRUCTIONS

1. Cut pork chops into bite sized pieces.

2. Coat in oil & seasonings.

3. Air fry for 10 minutes at 400F shaking the basket halfway through.

4. Take out, let cool, & enjoy!

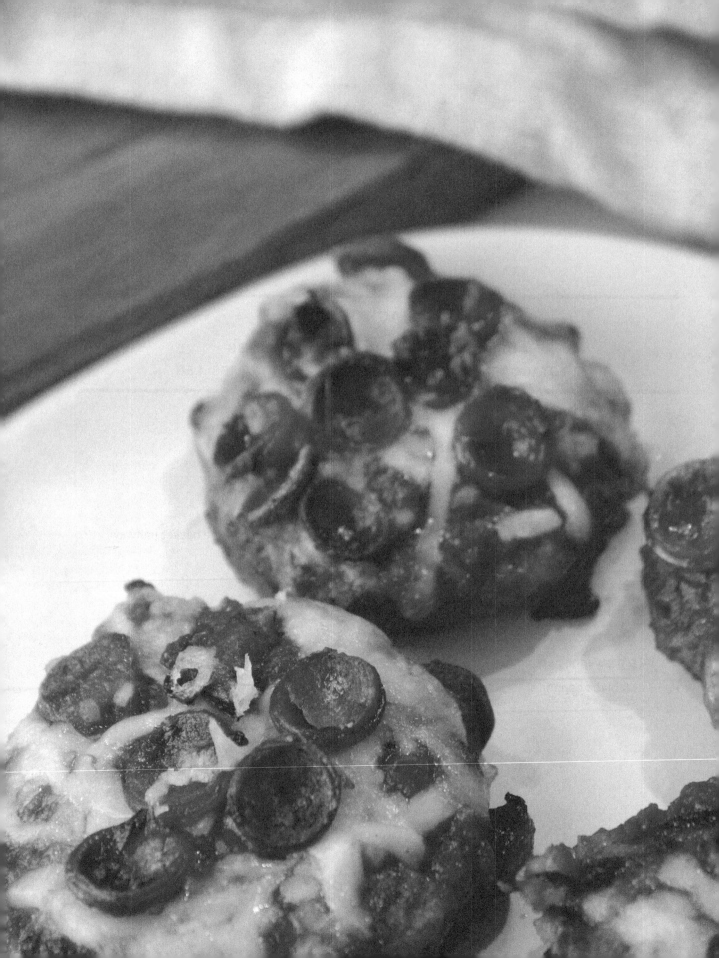

Sausage Crust Pizza Bites

RECIPE MAKES
1 SERVING

MACROS

◆ CAL: 680   ◯ FAT: 56G   ◠ PROTEIN: 42G

🌾 TOTAL CARBS: 7G   🍃 FIBER: 1G   🌾 NET CARBS: 6G

INGREDIENTS

- 4 sausage patties (fully cooked)
- ¼ cup marinara sauce
- ½ cup shredded mozzarella
- 16 mini pepperoni slices
- ½ tsp oregano

INSTRUCTIONS

1. Preheat the oven to 400F.
2. Warm up your sausage in the microwave for 30 seconds & add to a parchment lined dish.
3. Season and top sausage patties with remaining ingredients.
4. Bake for 15 minutes or until the cheese melts.
5. Take out, let cool & enjoy!

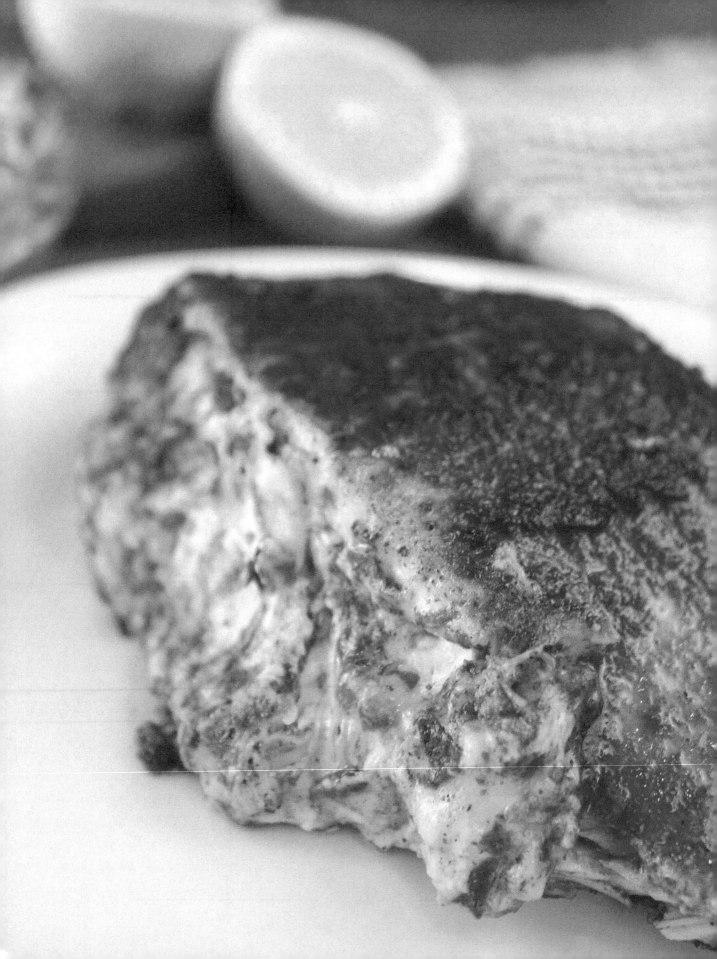

Stuffed Salmon

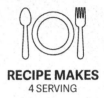

RECIPE MAKES
4 SERVING

MACROS

🔥 CAL: 352   🔥 FAT: 34G   🍳 PROTEIN: 38G

🌾 TOTAL CARBS: 2G   🍃 FIBER: 0.2G   🌾 NET CARBS: 1.8G

INGREDIENTS

- 4 Salmon filets
- 4 oz cream cheese
- 1 cup fresh spinach, chopped
- 1/2 cup parmesan
- 1/4 cup shredded mozzarella
- 2 tsp minced garlic
- Paprika
- Salt & pepper
- Olive oil & butter

INSTRUCTIONS

1. Pat your salmon dry and cut a slit into the middle about 90% through.
2. Drizzle with the olive oil & seasonings.
3. Combine remaining ingredients except butter into a bowl.
4. Stuff it into the salmon filets.
5. Add butter to a pan on medium high heat.
6. Add salmon filets to the pan for 6 minutes on each side.
7. Take off, let cool & enjoy!

Notes:

The amount of olive oil & butter will depend on how fatty your salmon is. Farm raised salmon will require less oil than wild caught sockeye salmon

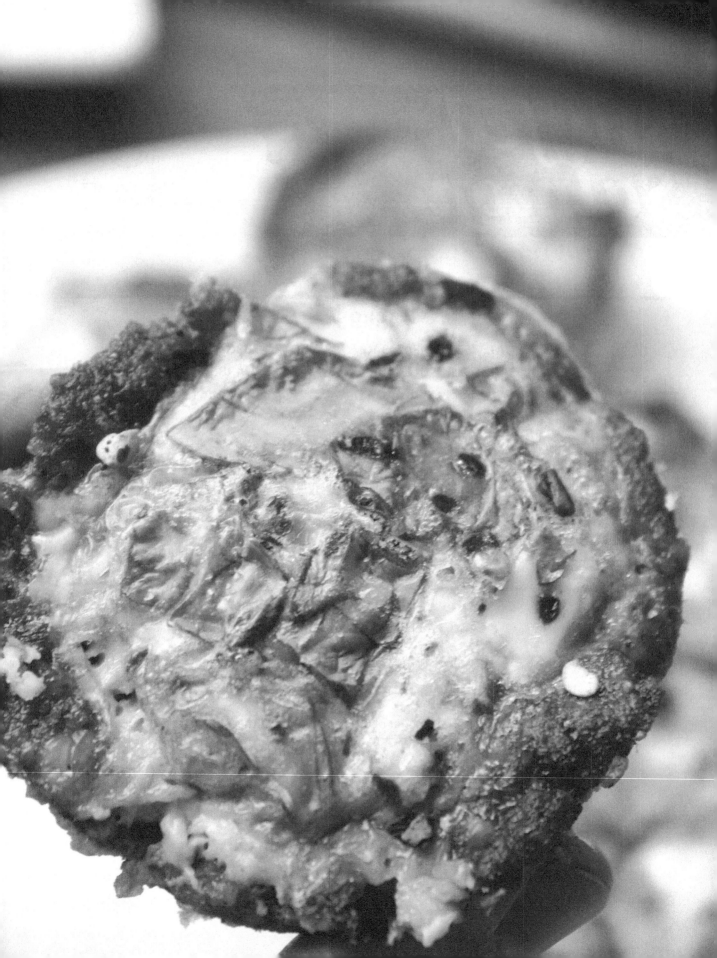

Spinach Feta Breakfast Cups

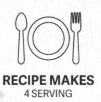

RECIPE MAKES
4 SERVING

MACROS

CAL: 302   FAT: 24G   PROTEIN: 14G

TOTAL CARBS: 2G   FIBER: 0.5G   NET CARBS: 1.5G

INGREDIENTS

- 12 oz ground sausage
- 3 eggs, whisked
- 1/2 cup fresh spinach, chopped
- 2 oz crumbled feta
- Red pepper flakes

INSTRUCTIONS

1. Preheat the oven to 325F.

2. Pat your sausage into 12 Patties, put them in a muffin tin and press down in the middle of each cup shaping it to the sides.

3. Combine remaining ingredients & add to your sausage cups.

4. Bake for 30 minutes, draining halfway through.

5. Take out, let cool & enjoy!

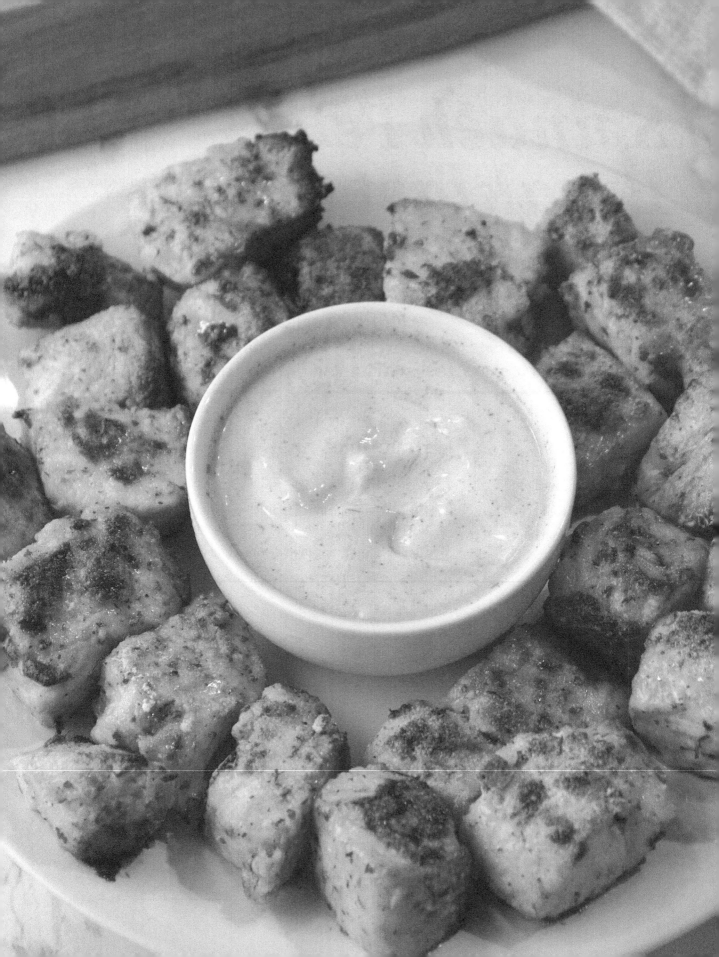

Salmon Bites

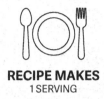

RECIPE MAKES
1 SERVING

MACROS (For 1/2 recipe, sauce not included)

🔥 CAL: 353   ⬤ FAT: 22G   🍥 PROTEIN: 38G

🌾 TOTAL CARBS: 1G   🍃 FIBER: 0G   🌾 NET CARBS: 1G

INGREDIENTS

- 1 lb salmon
- 3 tbsp butter
- 2-4 tsp chili lime seasoning

INSTRUCTIONS

1. Remove the skin from your salmon, pouring boiling water on it helps it come off easier!

2. Cut into bite sized pieces.

3. Melt your butter in a large bowl.

4. Mix salmon pieces & chili lime seasoning into the bowl with the melted butter.

5. Air fry at 400F for 10 mins, flipping halfway.

6. Take out, let cool & enjoy!

For the sauce:

1. Just mix 1/4 cup mayo with 2 tbsp sriracha!

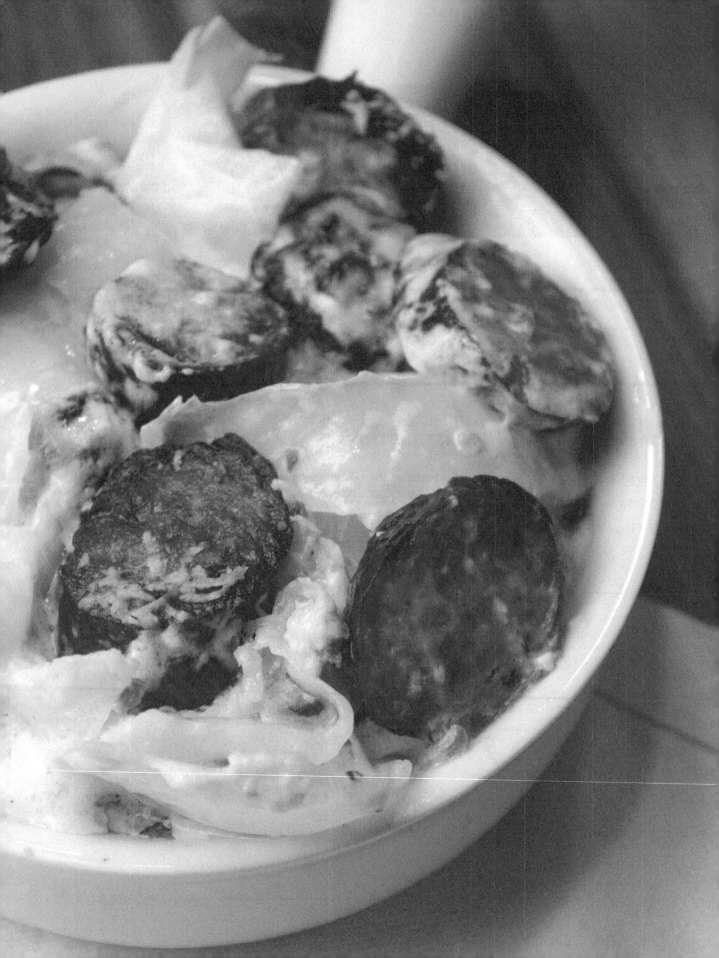

Sausage Cabbage Alfredo

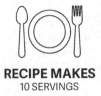

RECIPE MAKES
10 SERVINGS

MACROS

🔥 **CAL: 572**   🥑 **FAT: 52G**   🍳 **PROTEIN: 19G**

🌾 **TOTAL CARBS: 6.8G**   🍃 **FIBER: 1.6G**   🌾 **NET CARBS: 5.2G**

INGREDIENTS

- 1 medium head of cabbage
- 1.5 lbs smoked sausage
- 1.5 cups heavy cream
- 6 oz cream cheese
- 3/4 cup butter
- 1/2 cup grated parmesan
- 1 tbsp minced garlic
- 1 tsp onion powder
- Salt & pepper

INSTRUCTIONS

1. In a baking dish combine all ingredients except sausage and parmesan. (This works best in a cast iron skillet)

2. Cover and bake at 400F for 30 minutes.

3. Brown sausage and set aside.

4. Take out the baking dish, add sausage and parmesan, put back in for 5-10 minutes.

5. Remove from oven, let cool, & enjoy!

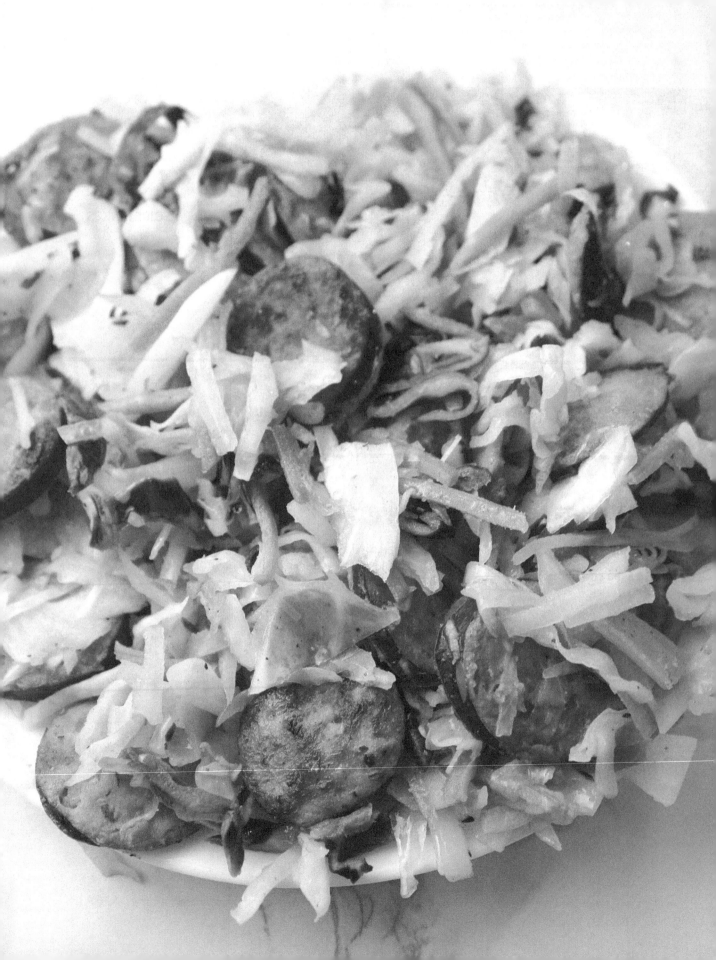

Sausage Slaw

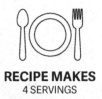

RECIPE MAKES
4 SERVINGS

MACROS

CAL: 404   **FAT: 36G**   **PROTEIN: 15G**

TOTAL CARBS: 5G   **FIBER: 1.3G**   **NET CARBS: 3.7G**

INGREDIENTS

- 16 oz fully cooked andouille sausage
- 4 cups cole slaw (undressed)
- 4 tbsp butter
- 1 tsp garlic powder
- 1 tsp paprika
- 1 tsp onion powder
- Salt & pepper

INSTRUCTIONS

1. In a pan on medium heat, brown your sausage.
2. Add the rest of your ingredients and stir until the cole slaw becomes tender.

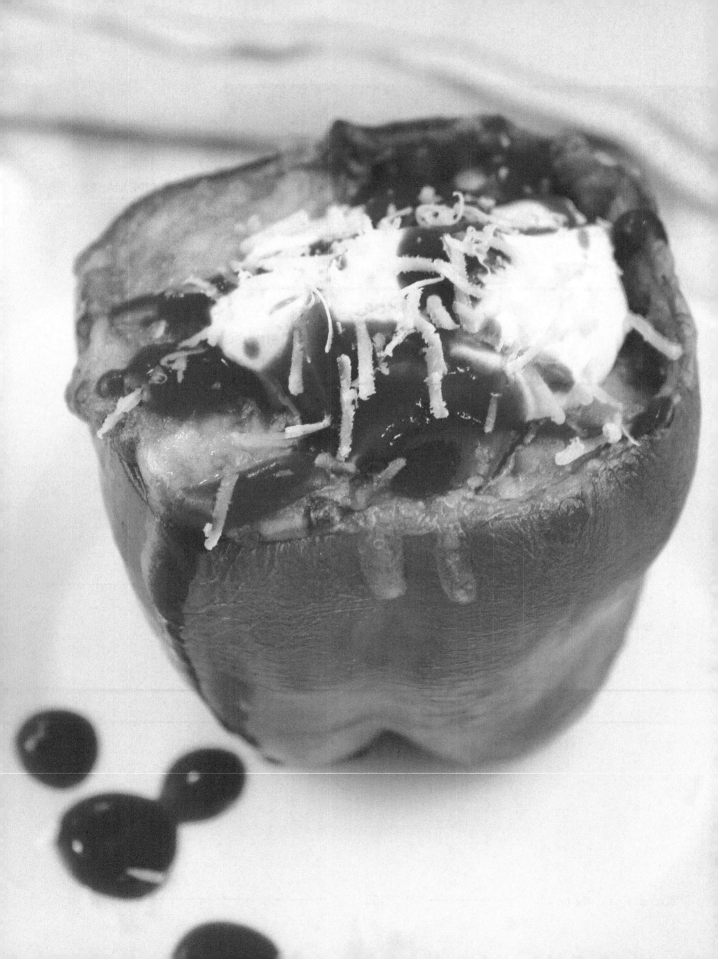

Sausage Stuffed Peppers

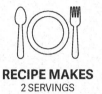

RECIPE MAKES
2 SERVINGS

MACROS

🔥 CAL: 489   💧 FAT: 37G   🍳 PROTEIN: 25G

🌾 TOTAL CARBS: 11G   🍃 FIBER: 3G   🌾 NET CARBS: 8G

INGREDIENTS

- 6 oz hot Italian sausage
- 3 oz cream cheese
- 3/4 cup shredded Mexican cheese
- 2 bell peppers
- Seasonings of your choice

INSTRUCTIONS

1. Cook your sausage and mix it with the cream cheese, 1/2 cup shredded cheese, and your seasonings.

2. Cut the tops off of your peppers and remove the insides.

3. Stuff your peppers and air fry at 360F for 6-8 minutes. Top with the rest of your cheese and put back in for 1-2 minutes.

4. Take out, let cool, & enjoy!

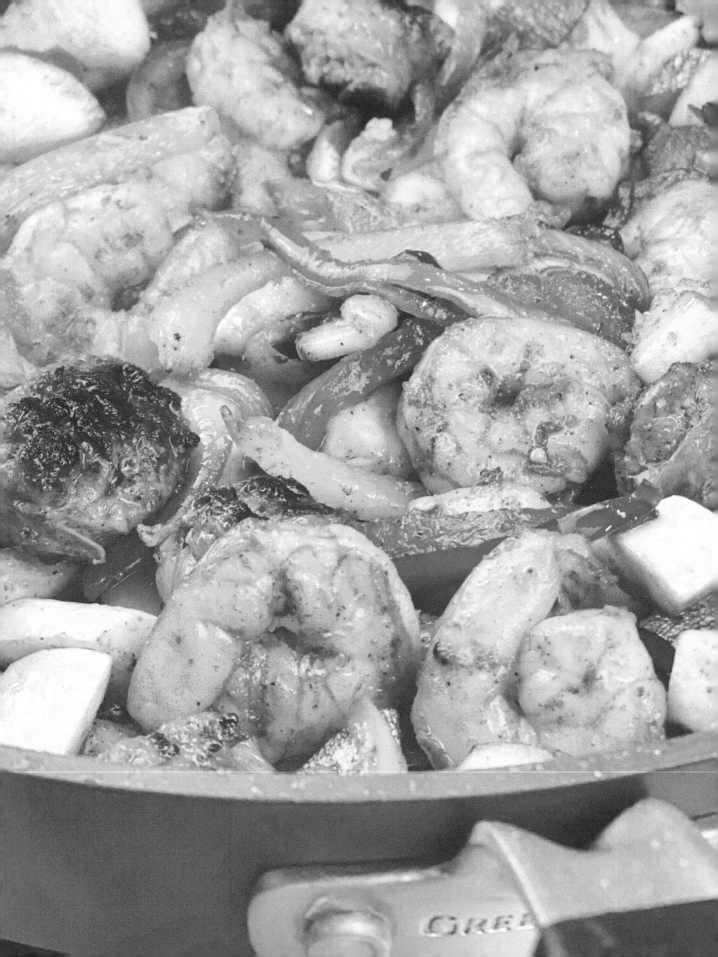

Shrimp & Sausage Skillet

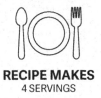

RECIPE MAKES
4 SERVINGS

MACROS

🔥 **CAL: 355**   💧 **FAT: 23.5G**   🦐 **PROTEIN: 28G**

🌾 **TOTAL CARBS: 6.5G**   🍃 **FIBER: 1.5G**   🌾 **NET CARBS: 5G**

INGREDIENTS

- 20 large shrimp, peeled and deveined
- 2 hot Italian sausage links
- 3-4 tbsp avocado oil
- 1/4 red bell pepper, sliced
- 1/4 orange bell pepper, sliced
- 1/4 yellow bell pepper, sliced
- 1 small zucchini, chopped
- 1 small yellow squash, chopped
- 1/4 red onion, diced
- 1 tbsp jalapeños, chopped
- 4 cloves garlic, minced
- 1/2 tsp garlic powder
- 1/2 tsp onion powder
- 1/2 tsp paprika
- Salt & pepper

INSTRUCTIONS

1. Pat dry shrimp and season to your preference.

2. Cook your sausage with 1 tbsp oil in a skillet over medium heat until browned. Remove and set aside.

3. Add 1 tbsp oil to your skillet on medium heat and cook the shrimp for 2 minutes on each side. Remove and set aside.

4. Add 1 tbsp oil to skillet on medium heat and cook your peppers and onions until translucent.

5. Add in the jalapeño, garlic, zucchini, squash, and seasonings and continue to cook for 5 minutes.

6. Add in the shrimp and sausage, stirring for 1 minute.

7. Remove and enjoy!

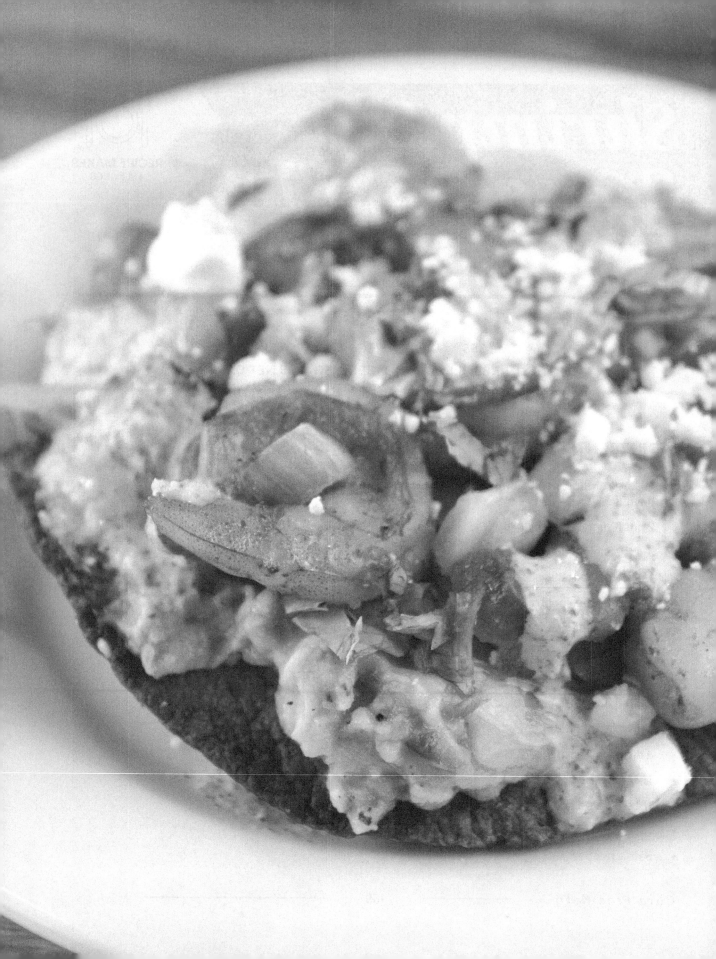

Shrimp Tostada

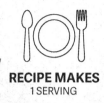

RECIPE MAKES
1 SERVING

MACROS

 CAL: 592   FAT: 52G   PROTEIN: 22G
 TOTAL CARBS: 18G   FIBER: 10G   NET CARBS: 5G

INGREDIENTS

- 1 low carb tortilla
- 6 large shrimp, peeled and deveined
- 1/4 cup shredded lettuce
- 3 tbsp guacamole
- 2 tbsp cotija cheese
- 2 tbsp diced tomatoes
- 2 tbsp diced red onion
- 1 tbsp chopped cilantro
- 1 tsp taco seasoning
- Salt & pepper
- Oil for frying

Optional:

- Aji Verde

INSTRUCTIONS

1. Fry your tortillas in hot oil until crispy on both sides. Or simply broil until crispy.

2. Coat your shrimp with salt, pepper, & taco seasoning.

3. Add to pan with oil over medium heat for 2 minutes on each side. Remove from pan & set aside.

4. Add all ingredients to the tortilla & enjoy!

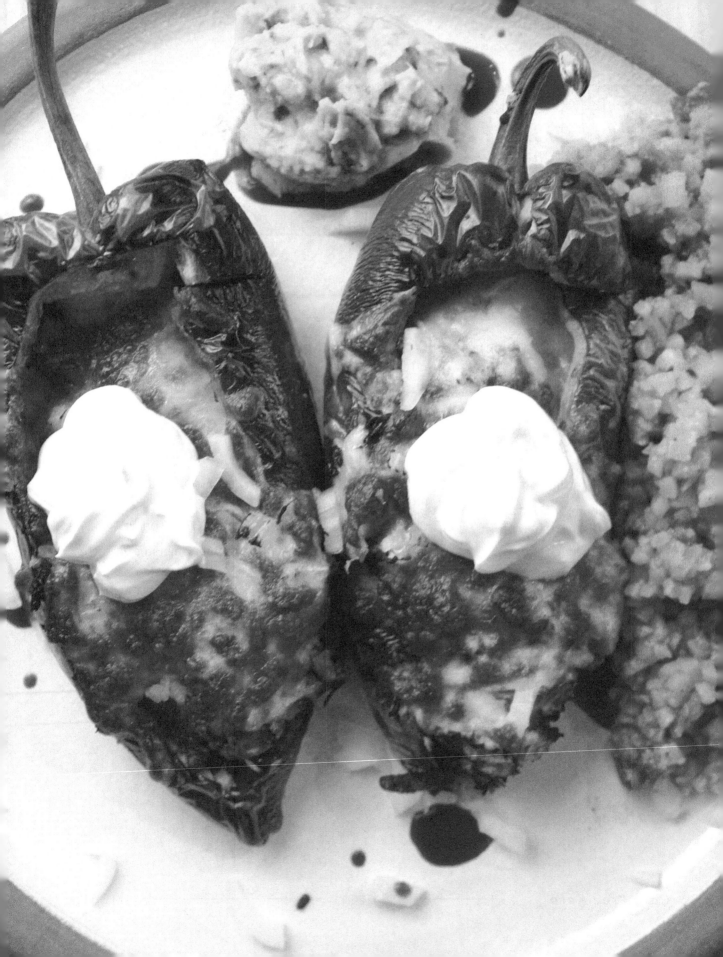

Stuffed Poblanos

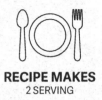

RECIPE MAKES
2 SERVING

MACROS

🔥 **CAL: 452**   🌢 **FAT: 31G**   🥑 **PROTEIN: 36G**

🌾 **TOTAL CARBS: 7G**   🍃 **FIBER: 2.5G**   🌾 **NET CARBS: 4.5G**

INGREDIENTS

- 1 poblano pepper
- 1/2 lb ground beef
- 1/2 cup shredded cheddar
- 1/2 cup frozen riced cauliflower
- 2 tbsp diced onions
- 2 tbsp sour cream
- 2 tbsp mild salsa
- 1 tsp cumin
- 1 tsp chili powder
- 1 tsp garlic powder
- Salt & pepper to taste

INSTRUCTIONS

1. Preheat the oven to 350F.
2. Slice pepper in half lengthwise.
3. Remove insides completely & bake on a greased baking sheet for 10 minutes.
4. Add ground beef, cauliflower rice, and seasonings to a large skillet and cook over medium heat for 5-8 minutes.
5. Remove peppers from the oven and stuff with cauliflower rice, beef, & onions. Top with cheddar.
6. Bake for 10 minutes until the cheese is melted.
7. Remove from the oven and top them with sour cream & salsa.

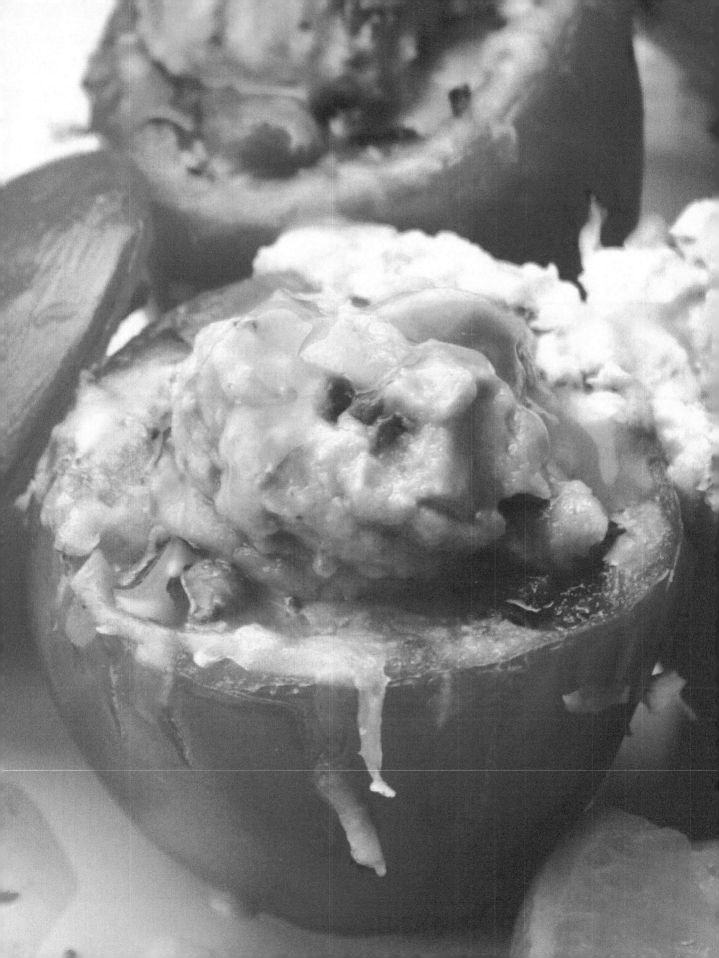

Stuffed Tomatoes

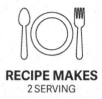

RECIPE MAKES
2 SERVING

MACROS

🔥 **CAL: 384**   🩸 **FAT: 31G**   🍳 **PROTEIN: 16G**

🌾 **TOTAL CARBS: 12G**   🍃 **FIBER: 2.8G**   🌾 **NET CARBS: 9.2G**

INGREDIENTS

- 4 medium sized tomatoes
- 8 oz pork chorizò (or ground meat of choice)
- 1 cup white onion, chopped
- 1/2 cup green chilies, chopped
- 1/4 cup cilantro, chopped
- 1 cup shredded cheddar
- 1/2 cup sour cream
- 1/4 cup guacamole or fresh avocado

INSTRUCTIONS

1. Preheat the oven to 350F.

2. Cut the tops off your tomatoes, hollow them out & pat the inside dry.

3. Add a tablespoon of cheddar, white onion, chorizo, and green chilis.

4. Repeat the above step.

5. Top with cheddar and sour cream.

6. Place tomato tops back on, add to the baking dish and bake for 25 minutes.

7. When done, add guac and your favorite hot sauce and enjoy!

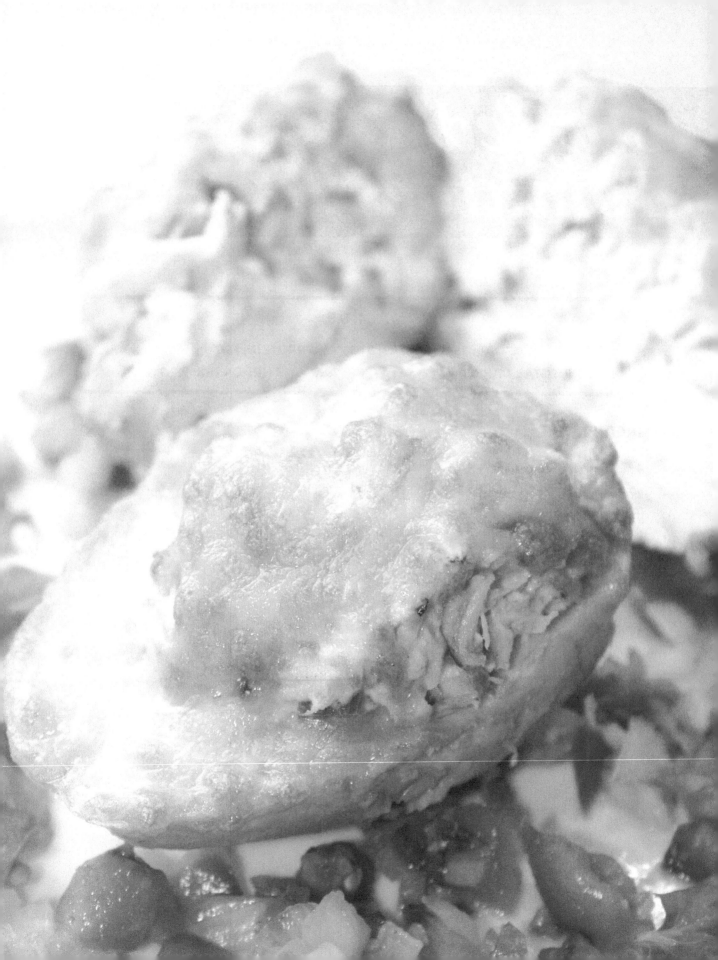

Tuna Avocado Boat

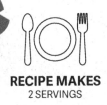

RECIPE MAKES
2 SERVINGS

MACROS

🔥 **CAL: 487**   🛢 **FAT: 39G**   🥑 **PROTEIN: 27G**

🌾 **TOTAL CARBS: 16G**   🍃 **FIBER: 10G**   🌾 **NET CARBS: 6G**

INGREDIENTS

- 2 large avocados
- 1/2 cup shredded cheddar
- 1 can of albacore tuna
- 1/4 cup red onion, chopped
- 1 tbsp cilantro, minced
- 1 celery stalk, diced
- 2 tbsp Mayo
- 1 tbsp Dijon mustard
- 1 tsp of fresh lime juice
- salt & pepper

INSTRUCTIONS

1. Preheat oven to 350F.
2. In a large bowl mix all ingredients except avocado and cheddar.
3. Slice avocados in half, peel the skin & remove the seed.
4. Add your tuna salad to the avocado & top with shredded cheddar.
5. Bake for 20-25 minutes.
6. Take out, let cool & enjoy!

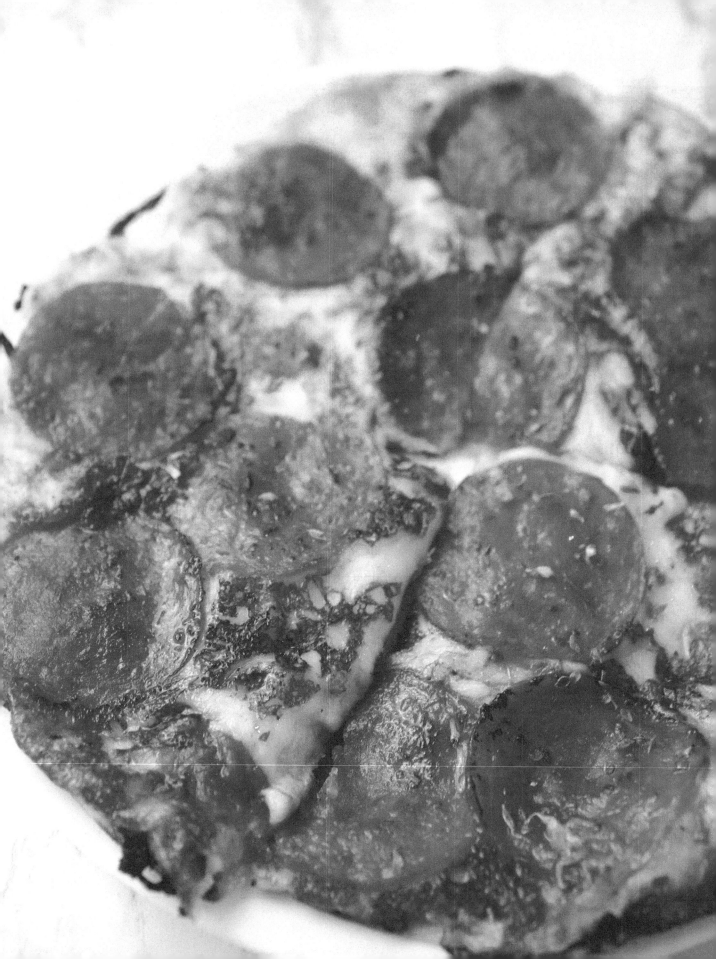

Upside Down Pizza

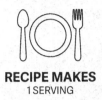

RECIPE MAKES
1 SERVING

MACROS

🔥 **CAL:** 450   🌢 **FAT:** 30G   🥚 **PROTEIN:** 27G

🌾 **TOTAL CARBS:** 24G   🍃 **FIBER:** 15G   🌾 **NET CARBS:** 9G

INGREDIENTS

- 10 slices pepperoni
- 3/4 cup shredded mozzarella
- 1/4 cup marinara sauce
- Low carb tortilla, 8-inch
- 1 tsp Italian seasonings
- salt & pepper

INSTRUCTIONS

1. Add pepperoni, mozzarella, & marinara to a non-stick pan on medium heat.

2. Top with low carb tortilla, after 2-3 minutes flip, and let the crust crisp up.

3. Season, remove from pan & enjoy!

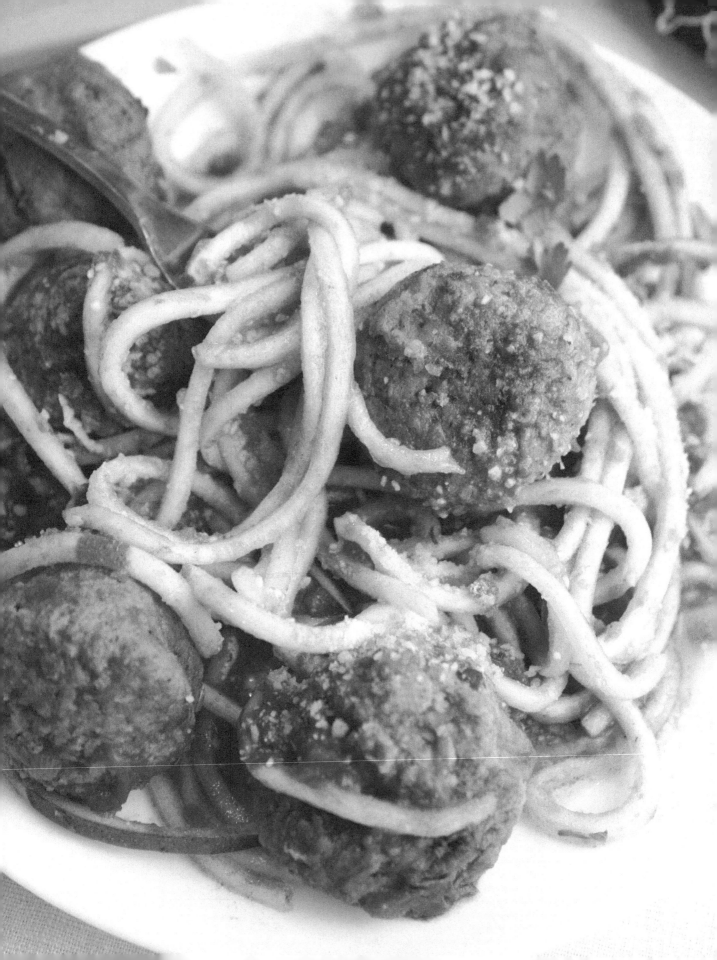

Zoodles & Meatballs

RECIPE MAKES
1 SERVING

MACROS

🔥 CAL: 419   🌢 FAT: 27G   🫛 PROTEIN: 37G

🌾 TOTAL CARBS: 11G   🍃 FIBER: 3G   🌾 NET CARBS: 8G

INGREDIENTS

- 4 fully cooked meatballs, frozen
- 1/2 medium zucchini
- 1/2 cup marinara sauce
- 1/4 cup grated parmesan
- 1 tsp italian seasonings
- salt & pepper

INSTRUCTIONS

1. Spiralize your zucchini and add to a plate uncooked.
2. Add your meatballs to a bowl and microwave according to the package.
3. Add your marinara sauce to the meatballs for the last 45 seconds in the microwave.
4. Stir well and pour over the Zoodles.
5. Top with parmesan and enjoy! Thank

Notes:

1. Macros will vary depending on the brand of meatballs used, but most Italian style meatballs in the frozen section will have around 4g net carbs for 4 meatballs.
2. You can cook the Zoodles if you prefer, but I enjoy simply letting the sauce warm them up so they keep their crunch.

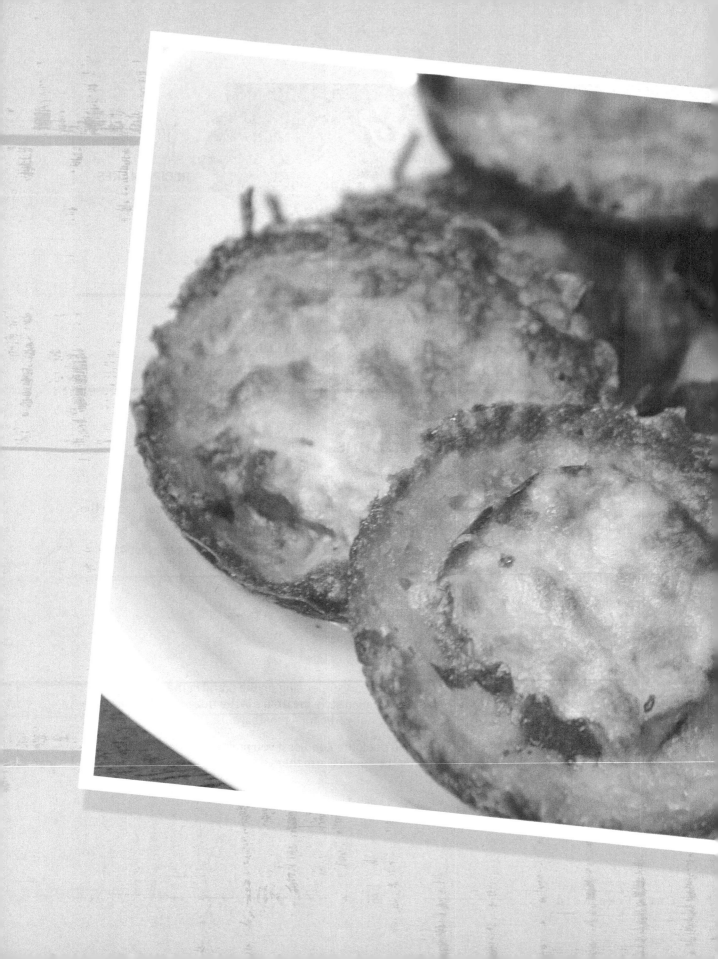

Snacks & Sides

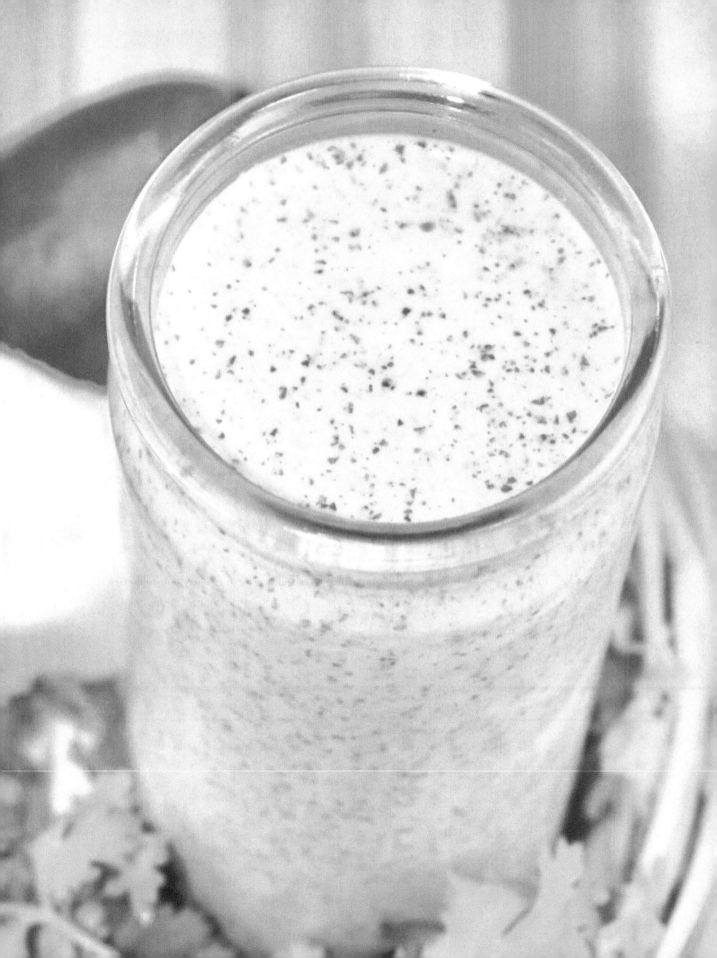

Aji Verde

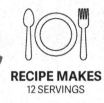

RECIPE MAKES
12 SERVINGS

MACROS

🔥 **CAL: 163** 💧 **FAT: 17G** 🥚 **PROTEIN: 0G**

🌾 **TOTAL CARBS: 1G** 🍃 **FIBER: 0G** 🌾 **NET CARBS: 1G**

INGREDIENTS

- 2 cups cilantro
- 3 jalapenos (take out seeds)
- 3 garlic cloves
- 1 cup mayonnaise
- 2 tbsp extra virgin olive oil
- ¼ cup parmesan cheese
- Juice of 1 large lime
- 1 tbsp white vinegar
- 1 tsp salt

INSTRUCTIONS

1. In a blender or food processor combine the cilantro, jalapenos, lime juice, parmesan cheese, garlic cloves, olive oil and white vinegar.

2. Blend ingredients well then add the mayonnaise and salt.

3. Blend again until smooth and creamy.

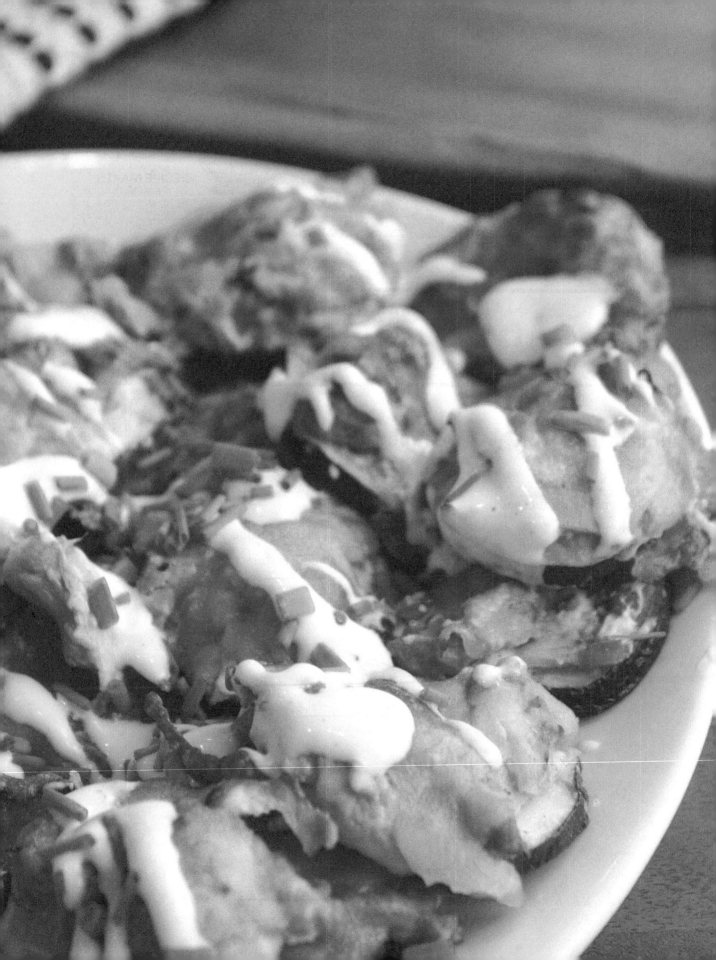

Buffalo Chicken Bites

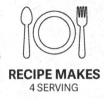

RECIPE MAKES
4 SERVING

MACROS

🔥 **CAL: 168**   🫗 **FAT: 12G**   🥩 **PROTEIN: 9G**

🌾 **TOTAL CARBS: 4G**   🍃 **FIBER: 0.5G**   🌾 **NET CARBS: 3.5G**

INGREDIENTS

- 1 medium zucchini
- 3/4 cup shredded chicken
- 3/4 shredded cheddar cheese
- 2 oz cream cheese
- 1/4 cup Buffalo sauce
- Salt & pepper

INSTRUCTIONS

1. Preheat the oven to 400F.
2. Slice your zucchini, pat both sides dry with a paper towel & salt heavily.
3. Combine remaining ingredients (except for 1/2 cup of your cheddar) & add on top of each zucchini slice.
4. Top with remaining cheddar.
5. Bake on parchment paper for 10-15 minutes. (Until cheese is golden brown)
6. Top with ranch, chives & anything else you enjoy!

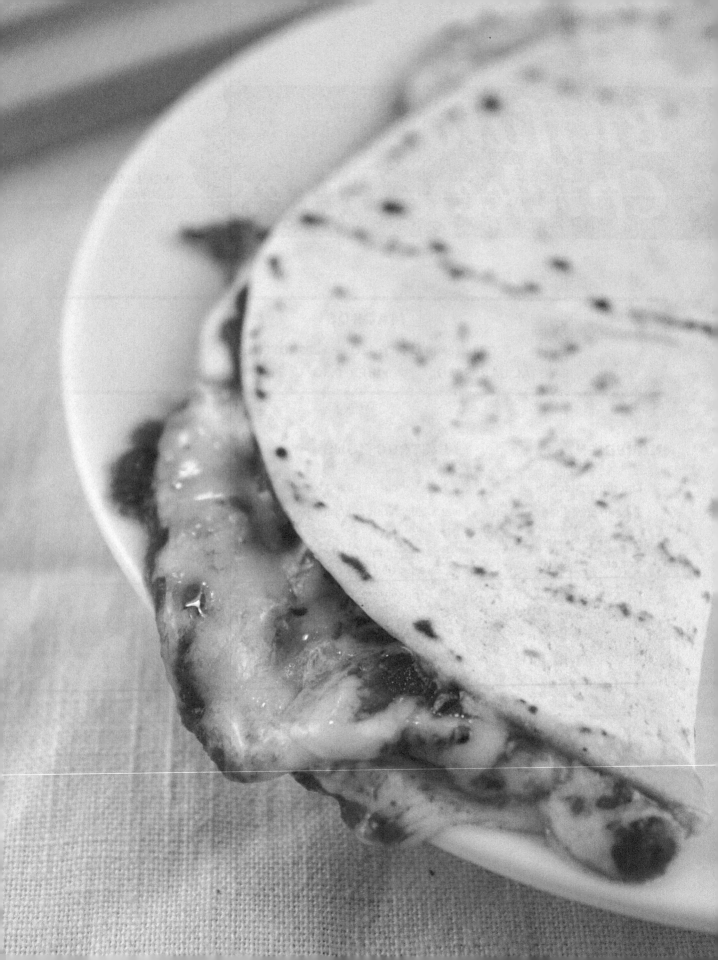

Bacon & Provolone Quesadilla

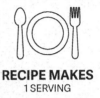

RECIPE MAKES
1 SERVING

MACROS

🔥 **CAL: 605**   ⬛ **FAT: 51G**   🥩 **PROTEIN: 26G**

🌾 **TOTAL CARBS: 25G**   🍃 **FIBER: 16.5G**   🌾 **NET CARBS: 8.5G**

INGREDIENTS

- 1 low carb tortilla
- 3 slices of bacon
- 1/2 cup shredded provolone & mozzarella
- 1/4 cup marinara sauce
- 2 tbsp sliced black olives (optional)
- 2 tbsp butter

INSTRUCTIONS

1. Cook bacon to your preference & chop.

2. Add butter to a pan on medium heat, coat your tortilla with the melted butter & remove from heat.

3. Layer half of your tortilla in this order - 1/2 of the provolone, bacon, seasonings, & the rest of your provolone.

4. Fold over and add back to the heat. Cook for 2-3 minutes on each side until golden brown and crispy.

5. Remove & enjoy!

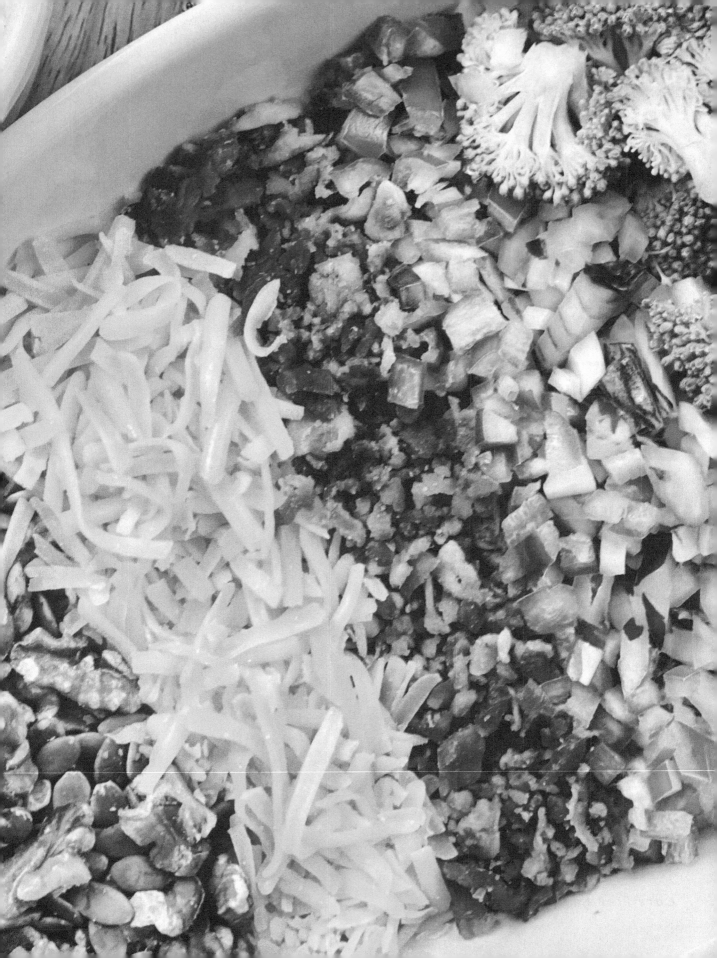

Broccoli Salad

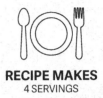

RECIPE MAKES
4 SERVINGS

MACROS

🔥 **CAL: 269**   ⬭ **FAT: 21.5G**   ⬭ **PROTEIN: 15G**

🌾 **TOTAL CARBS: 7.2G**   🍃 **FIBER: 2.7G**   🌾 **NET CARBS: 4.5G**

INGREDIENTS

Salad:

- 2 cups chopped broccoli
- 1/2 cup toasted walnuts
- 1/4 cup toasted pumpkin seeds
- 1/2 cup shredded cheddar cheese
- 1/2 cup bacon bits

- 1/2 cup chopped onion
- 1 chopped fresh jalapeño

Dressing:

- 1/2 cup sour cream
- 1 tbsp onion powder

- 1 tbsp garlic powder
- 1 tbsp apple cider vinegar
- 1 tsp salt
- 1 tsp pepper
- 1 tsp oregano
- 1 tsp sweetener
- 1 tsp fresh lime juice

INSTRUCTIONS

1. Combine all salad ingredients in a large dish.

2. Whisk together the ingredients for the dressing and drizzle over the salad. Enjoy!

Note:

You can blanch the broccoli in boiling water & toss into an ice bath if you don't like raw.

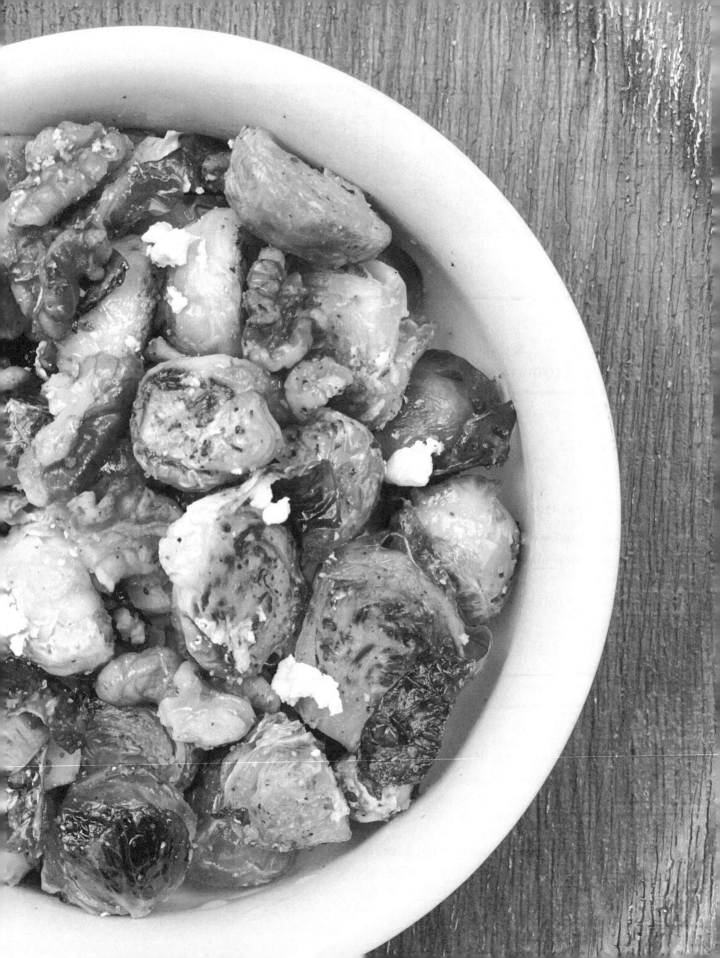

Balsamic Glazed Brussels Sprouts

RECIPE MAKES
4 SERVINGS

MACROS

🔥 CAL: 247   🛢 FAT: 21G   🥚 PROTEIN: 5.7G

🌾 TOTAL CARBS: 12G   🍃 FIBER: 4.8G   🌾 NET CARBS: 7.2G

INGREDIENTS

- 1 lb halved Brussels sprouts
- 1/2 cup toasted walnuts
- 3 tbsp extra virgin olive oil
- 3 tbsp balsamic glaze

INSTRUCTIONS

1. Preheat oven to 400F.
2. Toss Brussels sprouts with olive oil, salt, & pepper.
3. Add to baking sheet and roast for 20 minutes.
4. Remove from oven, add to serving dish and combine with walnuts and balsamic glaze. Enjoy!

Notes:

To make the glaze combine 1 cup balsamic vinegar with 1/4 cup allulose and bring to a boil over medium heat.

Reduce heat and simmer for 20 minutes until it reduces by 1/2.

Measure out desired amount & enjoy!

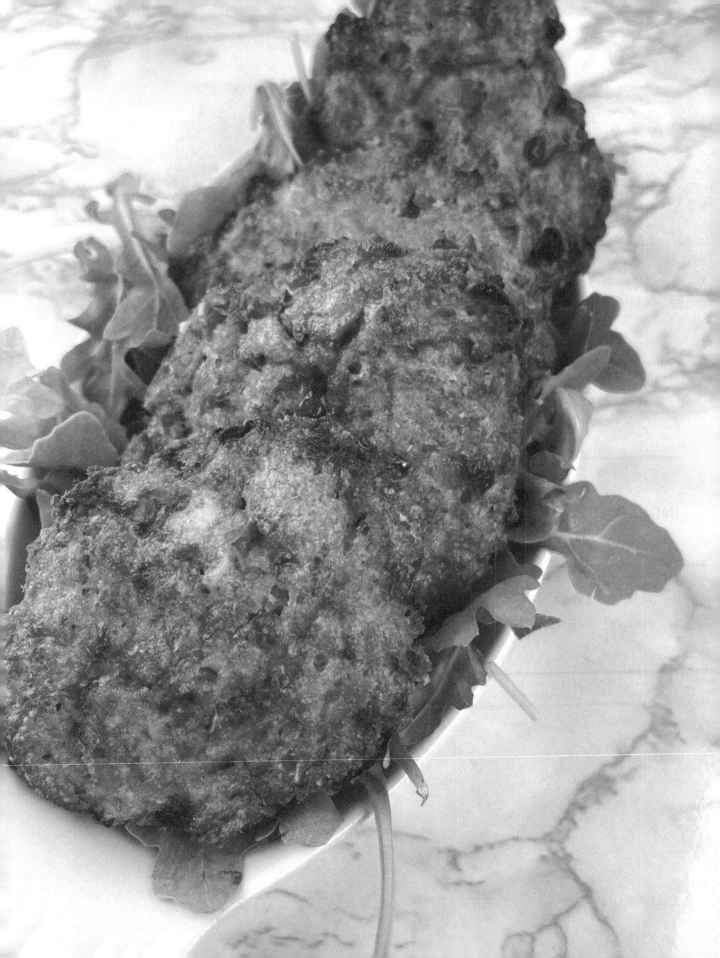

Crab Cakes

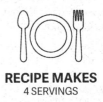

RECIPE MAKES
4 SERVINGS

MACROS

🔥 **CAL: 261**   🌢 **FAT: 25.1G**   🍳 **PROTEIN: 14.5G**

🌾 **TOTAL CARBS: 13G**   🍃 **FIBER: 6G**   🌾 **NET CARBS: 7G**

INGREDIENTS

- 8 oz lump crab
- 1/2 cup almond flour
- 1 large egg
- 1/4 cup chopped parsley
- 1 tbsp fresh minced garlic
- 1 tbsp Mayo
- 1 tbsp Dijon mustard
- 1/2 tsp salt
- 1/2 tsp thyme
- 1/8 tsp cayenne pepper
- 3 tbsp oil

INSTRUCTIONS

1. Whisk egg and mix with all ingredients except the crab, gently fold in the carb.
2. Shape into 8 patties and let refrigerate on wax paper for 1 hour.
3. Pan fry on medium until golden brown on both sides.
4. Let cool & enjoy!

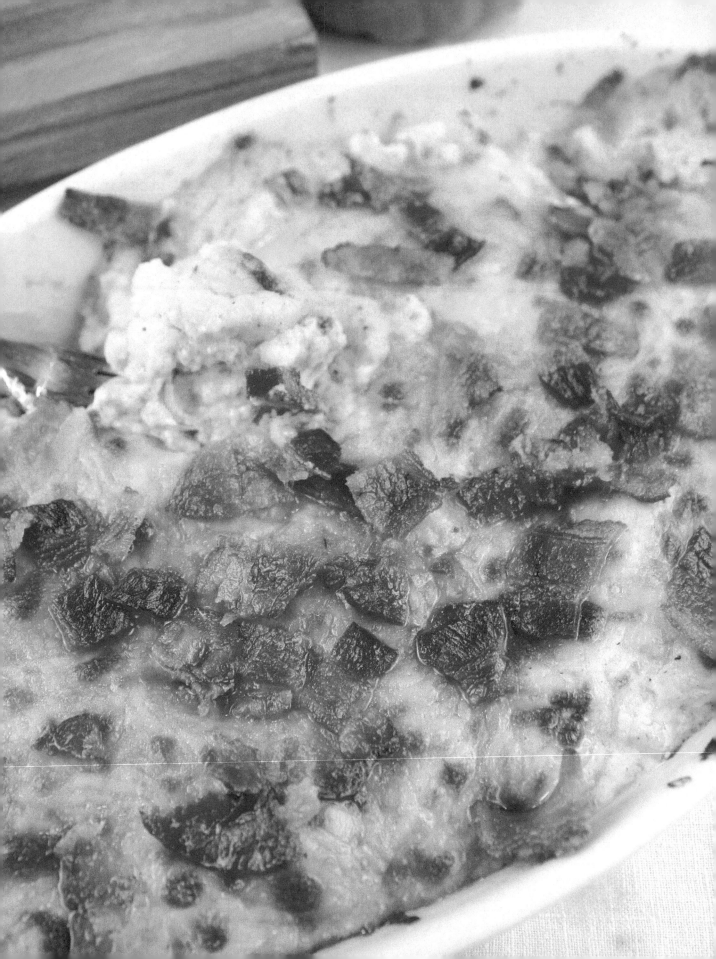

Cauliflower Mac & Cheese

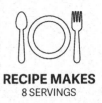

RECIPE MAKES
8 SERVINGS

MACROS

🔥 **CAL: 392**　　💧 **FAT: 35G**　　🥚 **PROTEIN: 14G**

🌾 **TOTAL CARBS: 7G**　　🍃 **FIBER: 2.5G**　　🌾 **NET CARBS: 4.5G**

INGREDIENTS

- 1 head cauliflower, cut into florets.
- 1 cup heavy cream
- 3 oz softened cream cheese
- 2 tbsp butter
- 2 tbsp olive oil
- 1 ½ tsp Italian seasonings
- 1 tsp garlic powder
- 1 tsp onion powder
- 1/ tsp chili powder
- Salt and pepper
- 2 cups shredded cheddar, divided
- 1 cup shredded Gouda (or cheese of choice)
- 1/2 cup bacon crumbles

INSTRUCTIONS

1. Preheat oven to 400F.
2. Coat cauliflower with olive oil, salt & pepper. Roast for 20 minutes and set aside.
3. Combine butter & cream cheese in a sauce pan over medium heat.
4. Add your seasonings, heavy cream, 1.5 cups shredded cheddar, & mozzarella to the pan and whisk until completely melted.
5. Add cauliflower to a greased baking dish and pour the sauce over your cauliflower.
6. Top with the rest of your cheddar cheese.
7. Bake at 400F for 20 minutes.
8. Remove from oven, top with bacon and fresh herbs for garnish. Enjoy!

Care Free Keto —————— **197** —————— SWEET TREATS

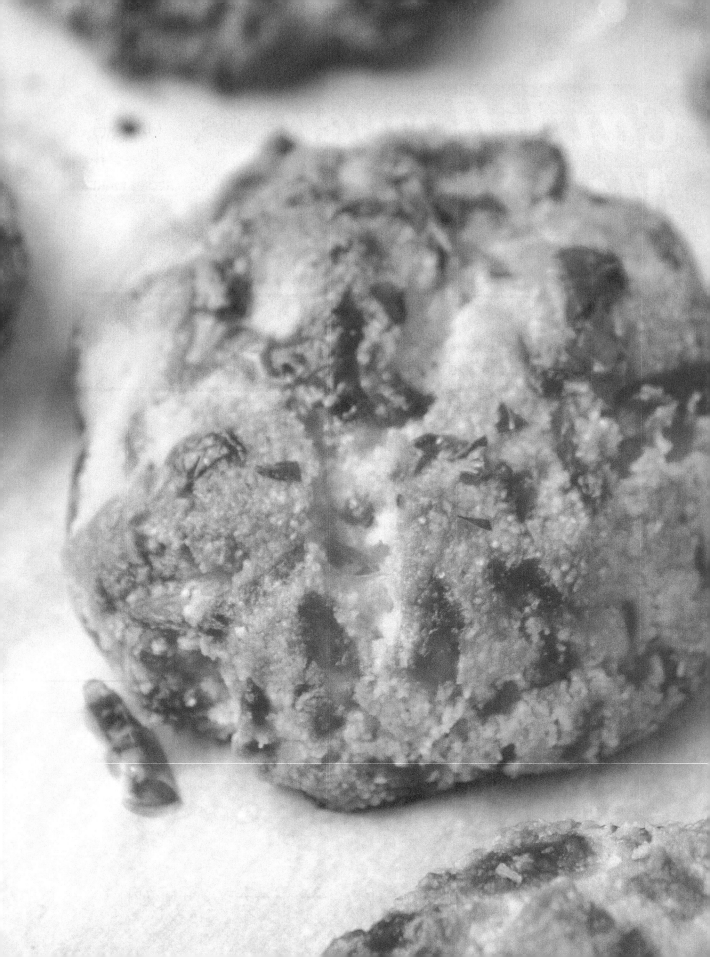

Cheddar Biscuits

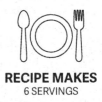

RECIPE MAKES
6 SERVINGS

MACROS

🔥 CAL: 493   💧 FAT: 47G   🍳 PROTEIN: 14.5G

🌾 TOTAL CARBS: 9G   🍃 FIBER: 4G   🌾 NET CARBS: 5G

INGREDIENTS

- 2 cups almond flour
- 2 tsp baking powder
- 2 tsp garlic powder
- 1/2 tsp salt
- 1 large Egg (whisked)
- 1/3 cup Heavy cream
- 1/3 cup butter
- 1 1/2 cup Cheddar cheese

Melted butter ingredients:

- 3 tbsp butter
- 1 tbsp Fresh parsley
- 1/4 tsp garlic powder
- 1/8 tsp salt

INSTRUCTIONS

1. Preheat the oven to 350F.
2. Melt butter & combine all ingredients except the cheddar.
3. Fold your cheddar into the mix & scoop out 12 balls on a parchment lined baking sheet.
4. Bake for 15 minutes (until golden). Remove from oven and let them cool for 5-10 mins.
5. Stir together your melted butter mix, brush it on top and enjoy!

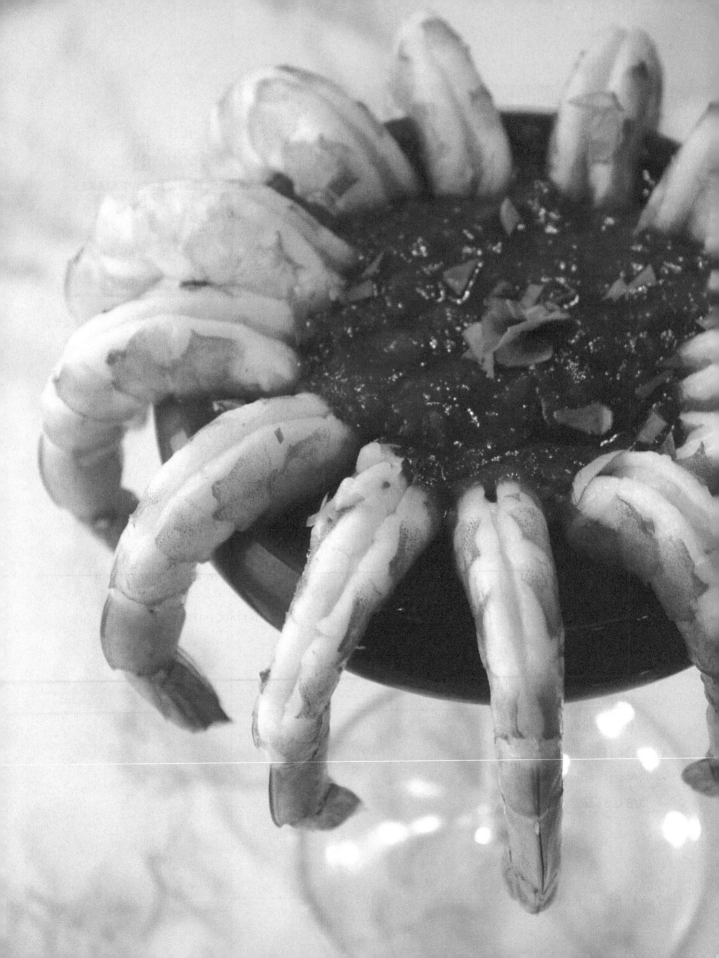

Cocktail Sauce

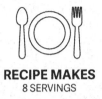

RECIPE MAKES
8 SERVINGS

MACROS

🔥 **CAL: 15**   🛢 **FAT: 0G**   🥚 **PROTEIN: 0G**

🌾 **TOTAL CARBS: 3.3G**   🍃 **FIBER: 0.5G**   🌾 **NET CARBS: 2.8G**

INGREDIENTS

- 1 cup sugar free ketchup
- ⅓ cup horseradish
- ½ tbsp worcestershire sauce
- 2 tbsp lemon juice
- ¼ tsp hot sauce

INSTRUCTIONS

1. Combine all ingredients in a blender and mix well.

2. Serve chilled with seafood of your choice.

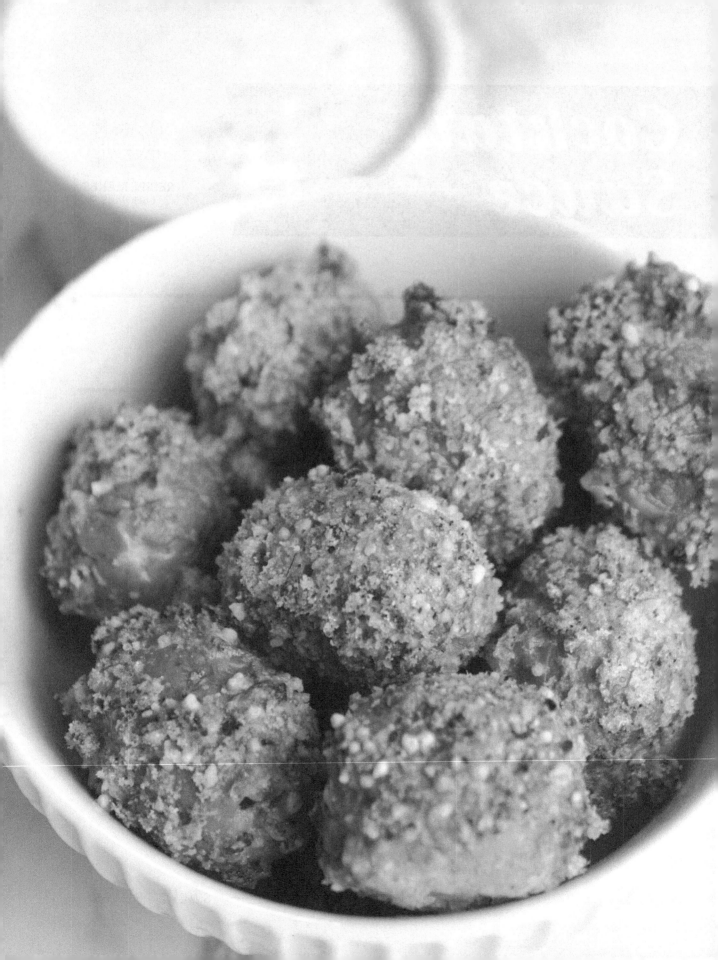

Cheese Stuffed Fried Olives

RECIPE MAKES
2 SERVINGS

MACROS

🔥 CAL: 385 🛢 FAT: 28G 🥩 PROTEIN: 32G

🌾 TOTAL CARBS: 1G 🍃 FIBER: 0G 🌾 NET CARBS: 1G

INGREDIENTS

- 10 large olives, stuffed with blue cheese
- 1/2 cup crushed pork rinds
- 1/2 cup grated parmesan
- 1 large egg
- Seasonings of your choice

INSTRUCTIONS

1. Whisk egg in bowl.
2. In another bowl add the crushed pork rinds and grated parmesan.
3. Pat olives dry, coat in egg wash and then the pork rind mix.
4. Air fry at 400F for 7-8 minutes.
5. Dip in Aioli and enjoy!

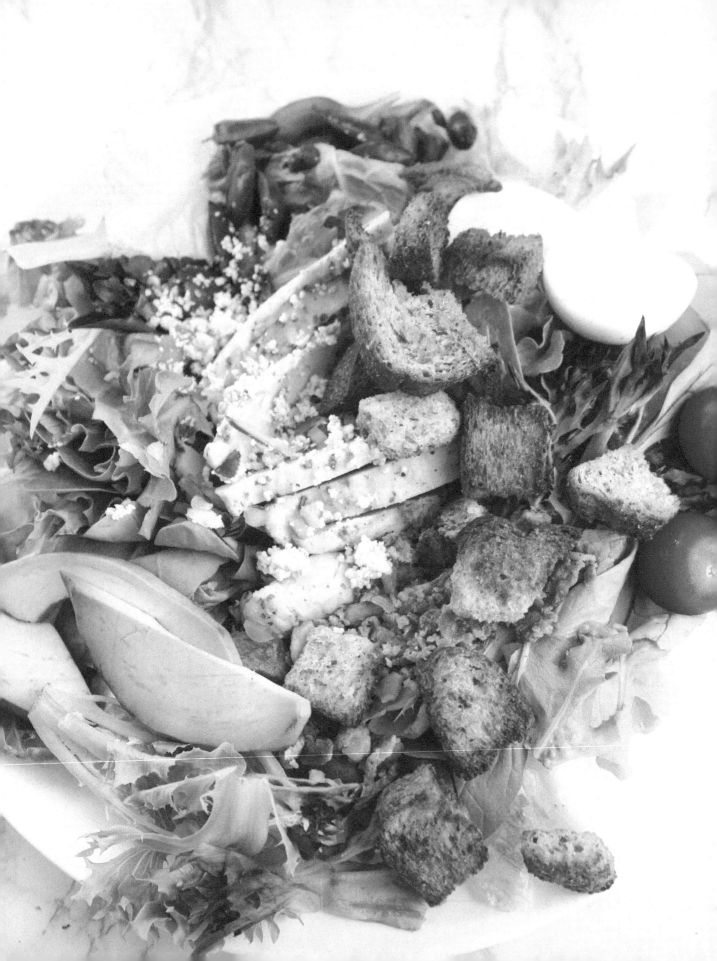

Croutons

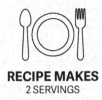

RECIPE MAKES
2 SERVINGS

MACROS

🔥 CAL: 172   🛢 FAT: 15G   🌱 PROTEIN: 5G

🌾 TOTAL CARBS: 7G   🍃 FIBER: 5G   🌿 NET CARBS: 2G

INGREDIENTS

- 2 slices low carb bread
- 2 tablespoons melted butter
- 1 teaspoon parsley
- 1/2 teaspoon onion powder
- 1/2 teaspoon seasoned salt
- 1/2 teaspoon garlic salt

INSTRUCTIONS

1. Cut up your bread into bite sized pieces.
2. Mix with all ingredients.
3. Air fry at 400F for 5-8 minutes!

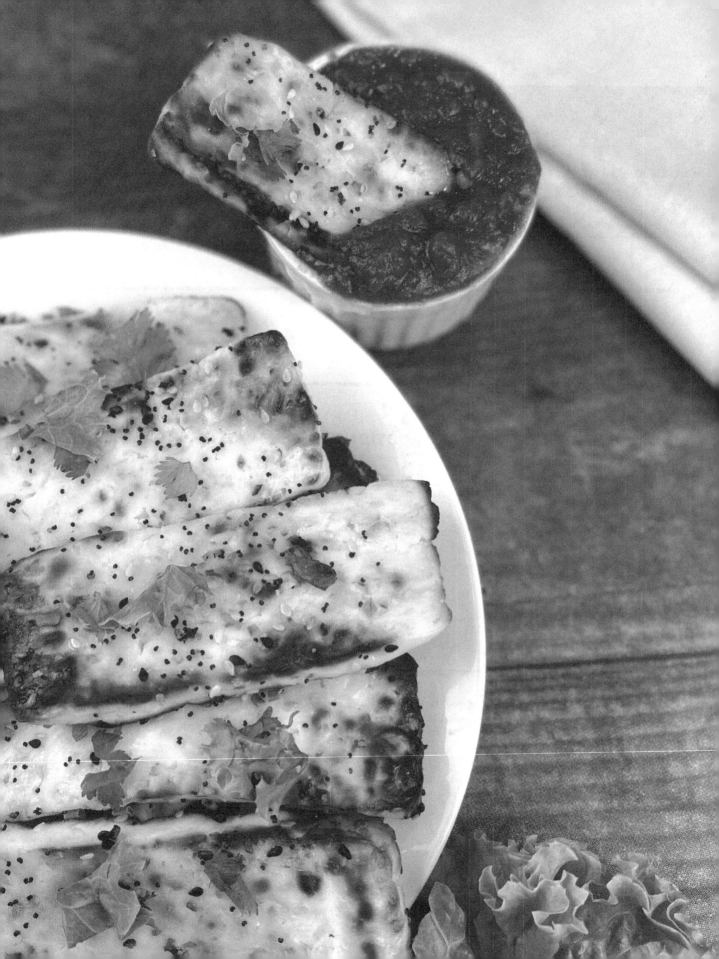

Cheesy Garlic Bread

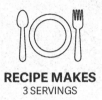

RECIPE MAKES
3 SERVINGS

MACROS

🔥 **CAL: 240**   🥑 **FAT: 18G**   🫘 **PROTEIN: 0G**

🌾 **TOTAL CARBS: 0G**   🍃 **FIBER: 18G**   🌾 **NET CARBS: 0G**

INGREDIENTS

- 1 block of Panela cheese
- 2 tsp everything but the bagel seasoning

INSTRUCTIONS

1. Slice cheese into 1/2 inch thick rectangles.

2. Season, add to parchment lined air fryer & cook at 400F for 6-8 minutes flipping halfway.

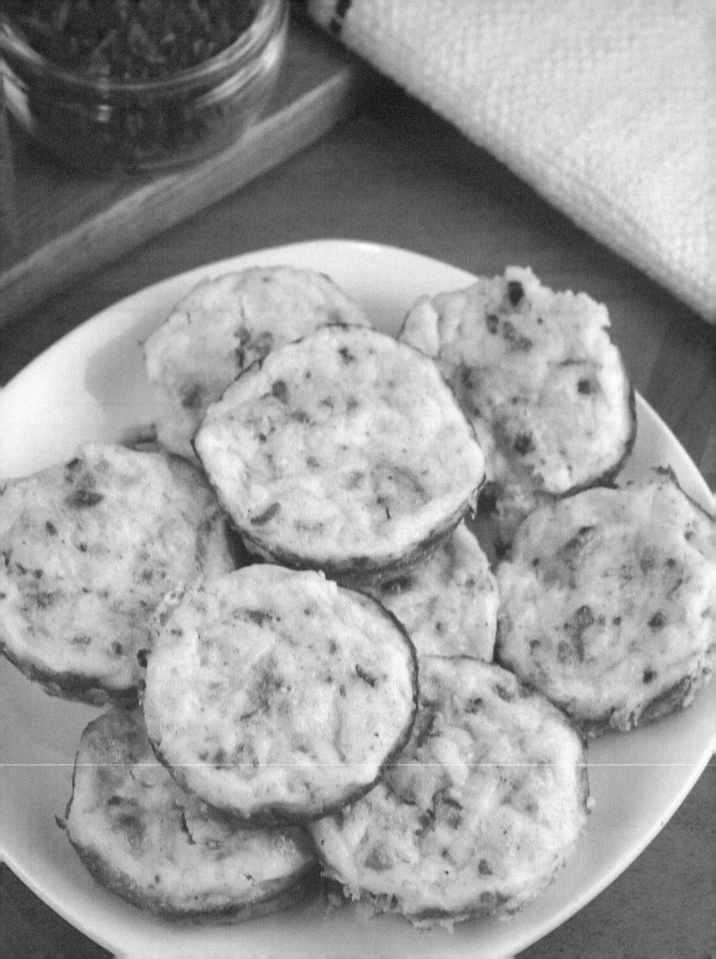

Egg Bites

RECIPE MAKES
4 SERVING

MACROS

🔥 CAL: 233   🛢 FAT: 16G   🥚 PROTEIN: 20G

🌾 TOTAL CARBS: 2G   🍃 FIBER: 0G   🥄 NET CARBS: 2G

INGREDIENTS

- 4 large eggs
- 1 cup cottage cheese
- 1 cup shredded Swiss & Gruyère
- Bacon crumbles
- Salt & pepper

INSTRUCTIONS

1. Preheat the oven to 350F.
2. Whisk eggs in a large bowl.
3. Add your cottage cheese, shredded cheese, & seasonings, whisk again.
4. Mix in your bacon and add to a greased muffin tin. (fill halfway so the eggs can expand)
5. Bake for 30 minutes, take out, let cool & enjoy!

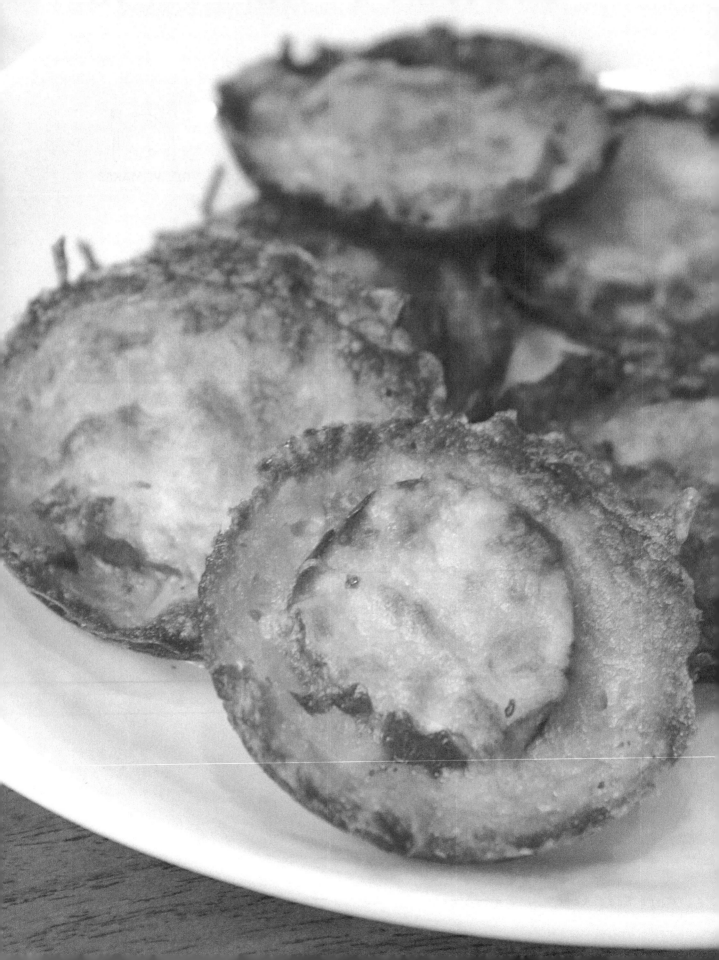

Fried Pickles

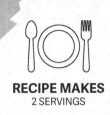

RECIPE MAKES
2 SERVINGS

MACROS

🔥 CAL: 208   🛢 FAT: 16G   🥚 PROTEIN: 14G

🌾 TOTAL CARBS: 2G   🍃 FIBER: 0G   🌾 NET CARBS: 2G

INGREDIENTS

- 1 cup shredded Mexican blend cheese
- 1/2 cup sliced pickles
- Seasonings of your choice

INSTRUCTIONS

1. Preheat oven to 400F.
2. Pat your pickles completely dry.
3. Add a small pile of cheese to each cup in a non-stick muffin tin.
4. Top with 1-2 pickles, the rest of your cheese, & bake for 20 minutes until the top begins to crisp up.
5. Remove from oven, let cool 10 minutes, & enjoy!

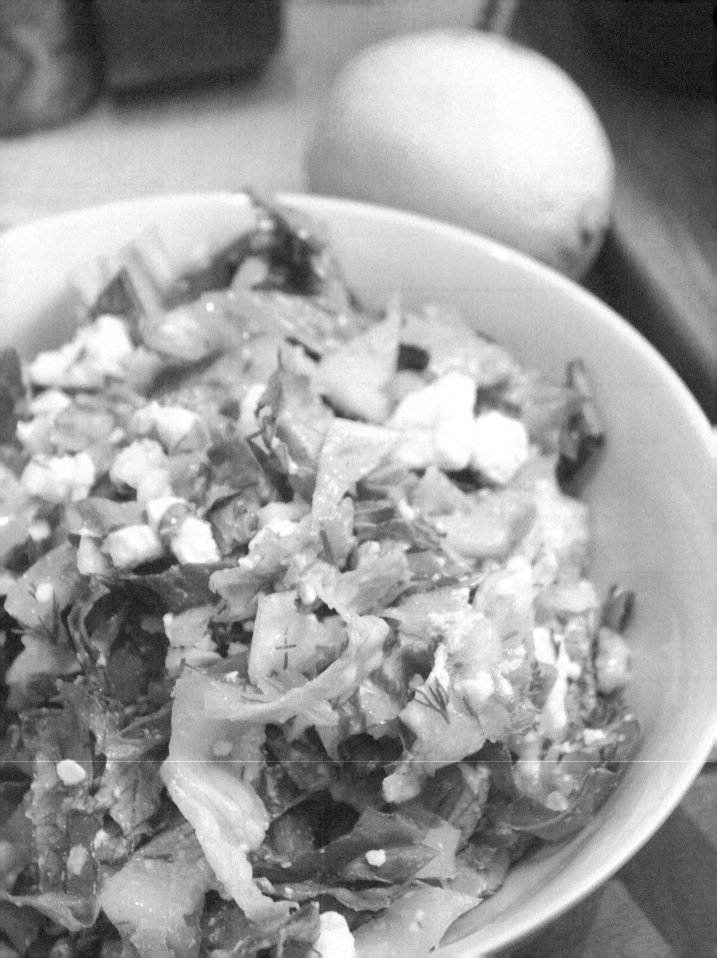

Greek Salad

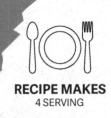

RECIPE MAKES
4 SERVING

MACROS

🜄 CAL: 119   🜄 FAT: 11G   🥢 PROTEIN: 2G

🌾 TOTAL CARBS: 7G   🌿 FIBER: 4G   🌾 NET CARBS: 3G

INGREDIENTS

- 3 cups chopped romaine
- 2 oz crumbled feta
- 1/2 cup shallots
- 1/4 cup fresh dill
- 2 tbsp olive oil
- Juice of 1/2 lemon

INSTRUCTIONS

1. Combine all ingredients except for olive oil, lemon juice & salt in a large bowl.

2. Whisk together remaining ingredients for your dressing & massage it into the salad.

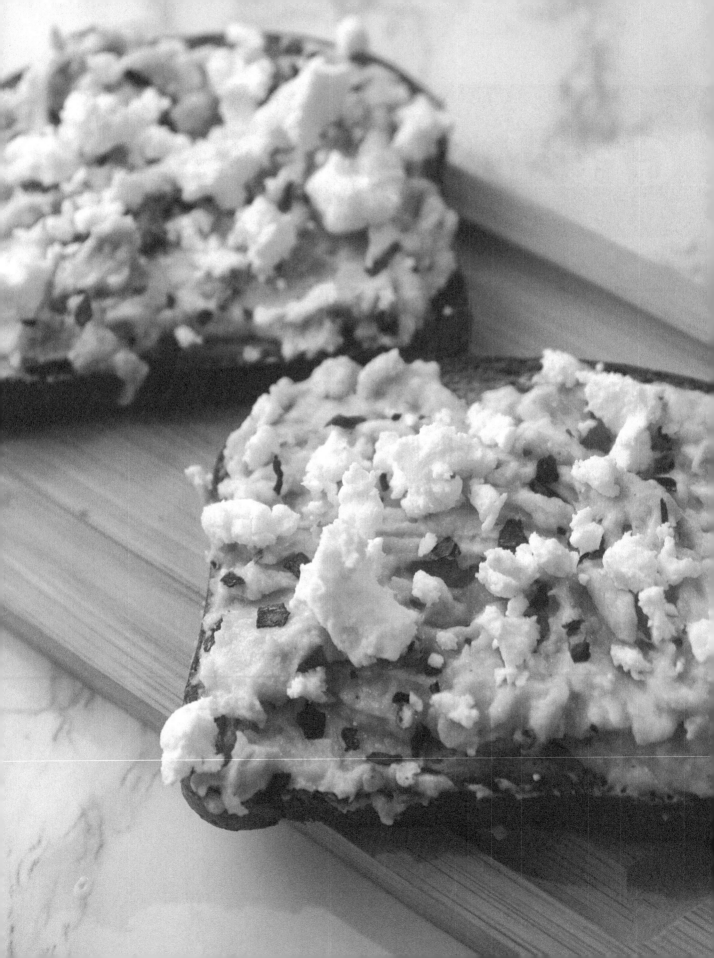

Goat Cheese Avocado Toast

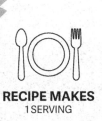

RECIPE MAKES
1 SERVING

MACROS

 CAL: 312   FAT: 25G   PROTEIN: 16G

 TOTAL CARBS: 12G   FIBER: 8G   NET CARBS: 4G

INGREDIENTS

- 1 slice low carb bread
- 3 tbsp avocado, mashed
- 2 tbsp goat cheese crumbles
- Red pepper flakes
- Salt & pepper

INSTRUCTIONS

1. Toast your slice of bread.

2. Add your avocado, goat cheese, & seasonings.

3. Enjoy!

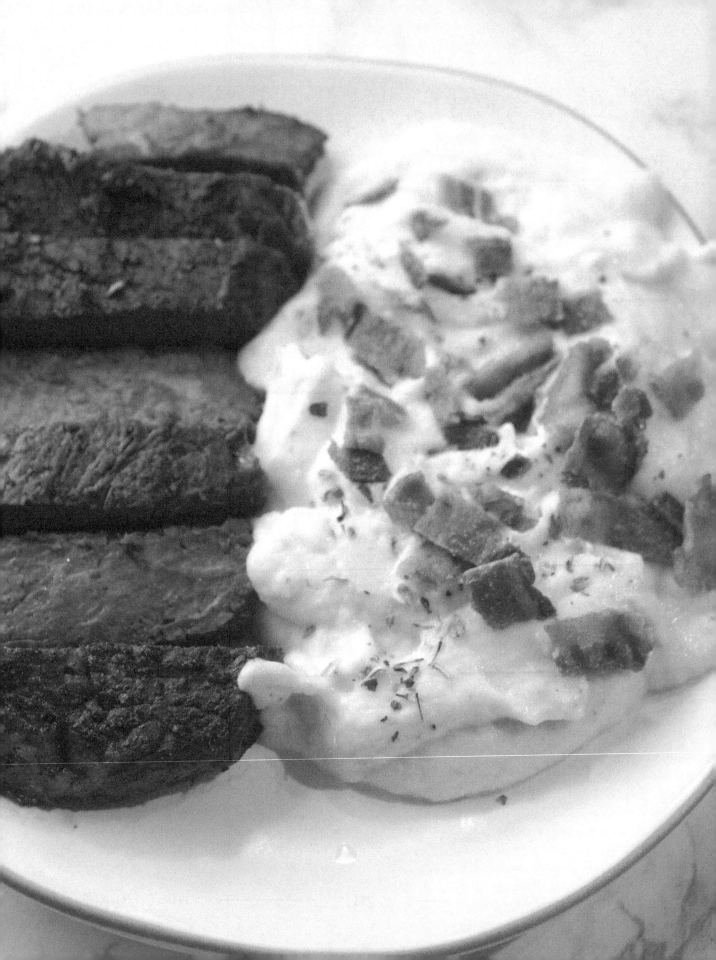

Mashed Cauliflower

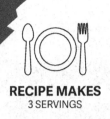

RECIPE MAKES
3 SERVINGS

MACROS

🔥 **CAL: 150**   🌢 **FAT: 11G**   🥚 **PROTEIN: 4G**

🌾 **TOTAL CARBS: 10G**   🍃 **FIBER: 3.6G**   🌾 **NET CARBS: 6.4G**

INGREDIENTS

- 1 Head of cauliflower
- 2 tbsp butter
- 2 tbsp cream cheese
- 2 cloves or garlic
- Salt & pepper

Optional:

- Shredded cheddar
- Bacon

INSTRUCTIONS

1. Chop your cauliflower head into florets & boil for 7-8 minutes.

2. Drain, add back to the heat for a few minutes & let it cook out the moisture.

3. Add to a blender with butter, cream cheese, shredded cheddar & seasonings.

4. Pour out, garnish, & enjoy!

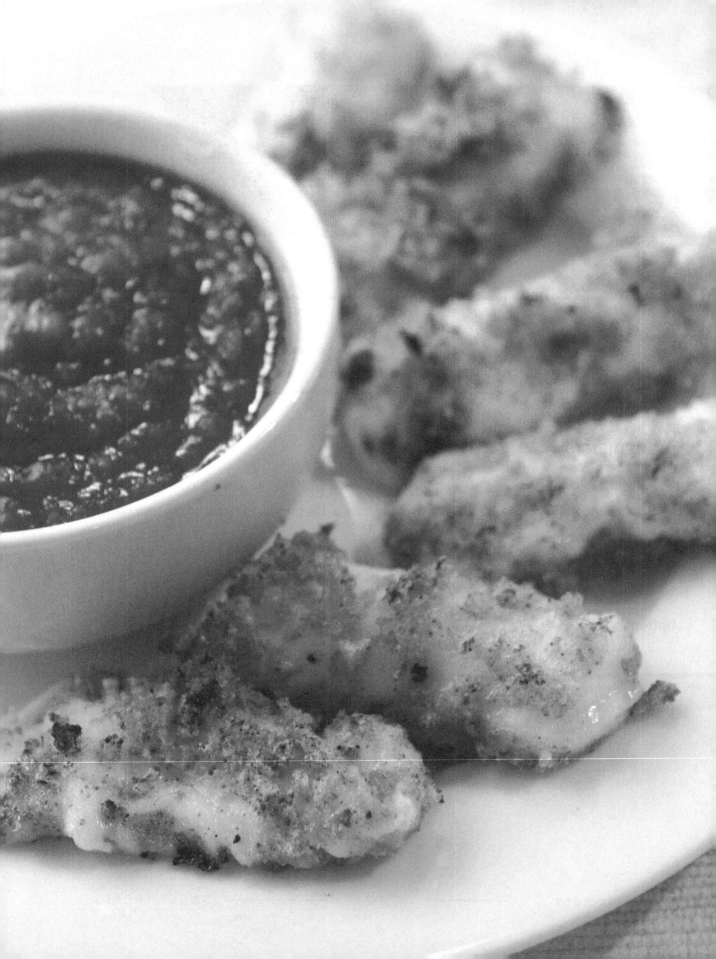

Mini Mozzarella Sticks

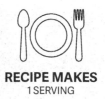

RECIPE MAKES
1 SERVING

MACROS

🔥 **CAL: 474**   🛢 **FAT: 30G**   🥚 **PROTEIN: 43G**

🌾 **TOTAL CARBS: 4G**   🍃 **FIBER: 0G**   🌾 **NET CARBS: 4G**

INGREDIENTS

- 4 mozzarella sticks, frozen
- 1 large egg, whisked
- 1 cup crushed pork rinds

INSTRUCTIONS

1. Cut mozzarella sticks in half.

2. Coat in egg and pork rinds.

3. Air fry at 400F for 5-10 minutes.

4. Take out, let cool, & enjoy!

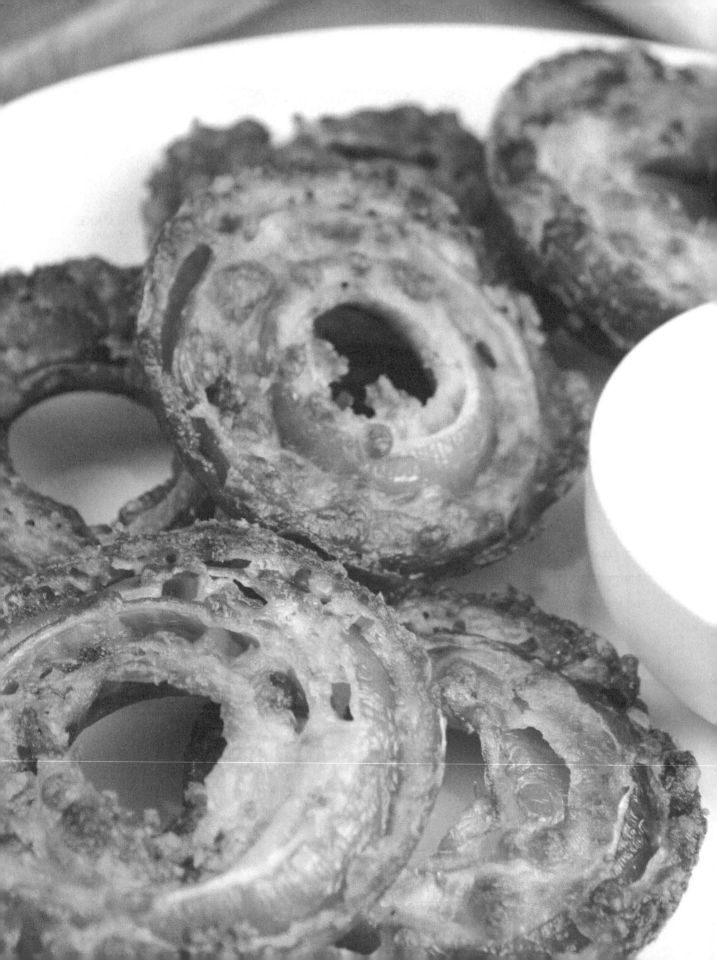

Onion Rings

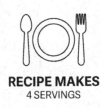

RECIPE MAKES
4 SERVINGS

MACROS

💧 CAL: 355   🔥 FAT: 27G   🥚 PROTEIN: 19G

🌾 TOTAL CARBS: 8G   🍃 FIBER: 1G   🌾 NET CARBS: 8G

INGREDIENTS

- 1 cup shredded Mexican cheese
- 1/3 cup sliced onions
- Chili powder
- Salt & pepper

INSTRUCTIONS

1. Preheat oven to 400F.
2. Add half of your cheese to a non-stick muffin tin or donut mold.
3. Top with sliced onions & cover completely with more cheese.
4. Season generously.
5. Bake for 15 minutes.
6. Let cool for 5-10 minutes and enjoy!

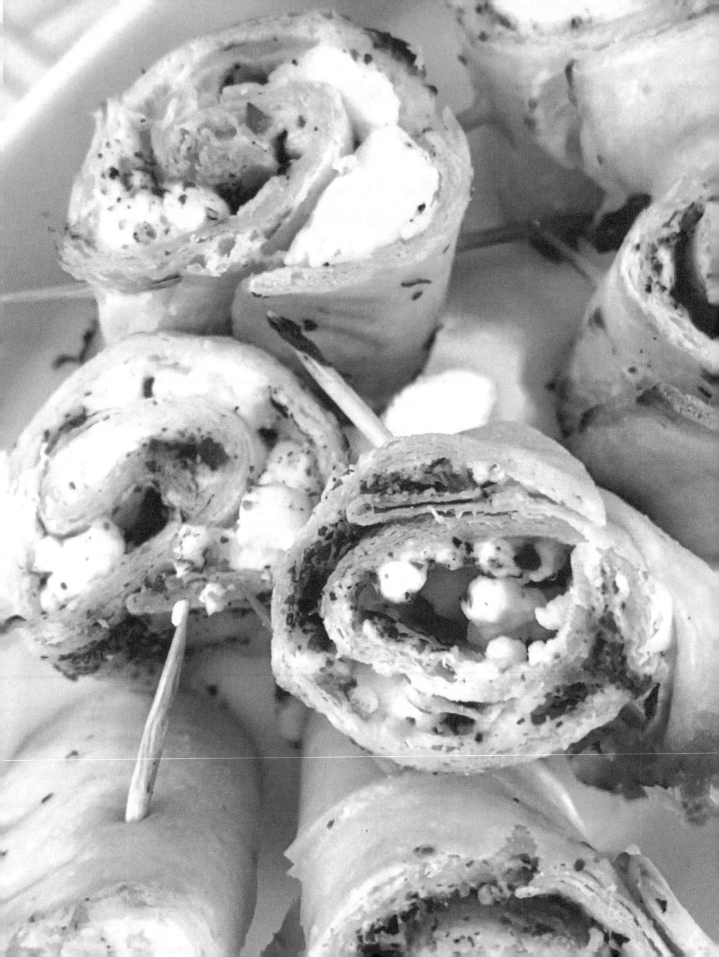

Pesto Roll Ups

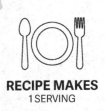

RECIPE MAKES
1 SERVING

MACROS

🔥 CAL: 484   🛢 FAT: 42G   🫘 PROTEIN: 21G

🌾 TOTAL CARBS: 21G   🍃 FIBER: 15G   🌾 NET CARBS: 6G

INGREDIENTS

- 1 tbsp cream cheese
- 1 tbsp butter
- 2 oz goat cheese
- 2 tbsp pesto
- Low carb tortilla, 8 inch
- Red pepper flakes
- Oregano
- Salt & pepper

INSTRUCTIONS

1. Spread ingredients on low carb tortilla.
2. Roll up and drizzle with melted butter & oregano.
3. Air fry at 400F for 7 minutes.
4. Take out, let cool, & enjoy!

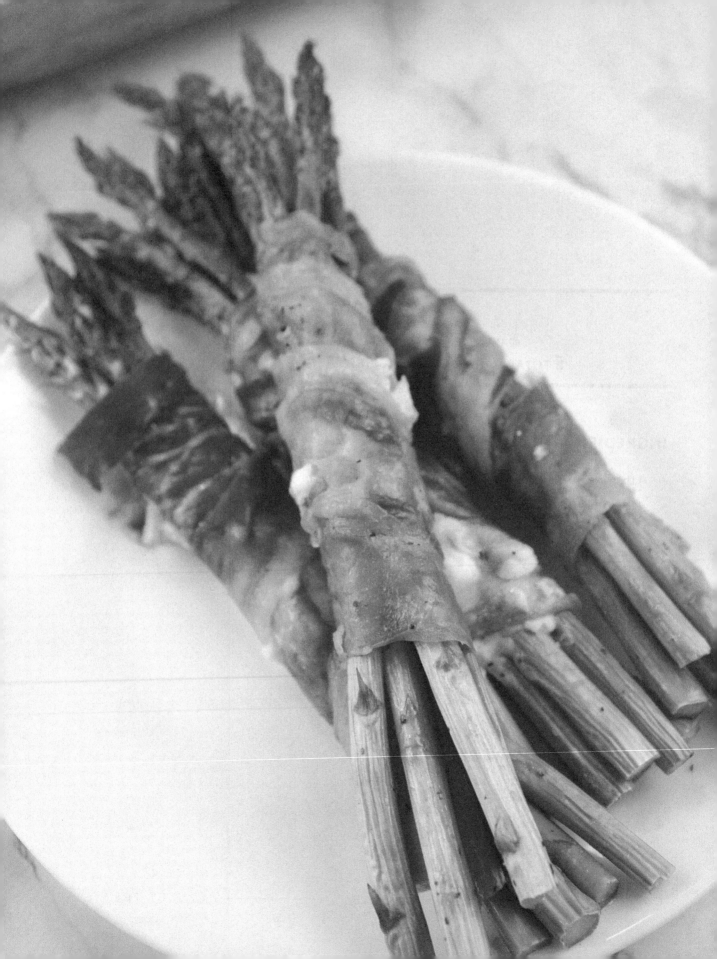

Prosciutto Wrapped Asparagus

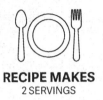

RECIPE MAKES
2 SERVINGS

MACROS

🔥 **CAL: 298**   🥑 **FAT: 22.5G**   🫛 **PROTEIN: 18G**

🌾 **TOTAL CARBS: 9.5G**   🍃 **FIBER: 4.5G**   🌾 **NET CARBS: 5G**

INGREDIENTS

- 3 oz prosciutto
- 1 lb. asparagus
- 3 tbsp cream cheese
- 2 tbsp olive oil
- Salt & pepper

INSTRUCTIONS

1. Preheat oven to 425F.
2. Rinse and cut the ends off of your asparagus.
3. Coat with olive oil and seasonings.
4. Separate your slices of prosciutto and spread cream cheese over them.
5. Divide asparagus into 4 bundles, wrap each bundle with prosciutto and bake for 8-12 minutes. Enjoy!

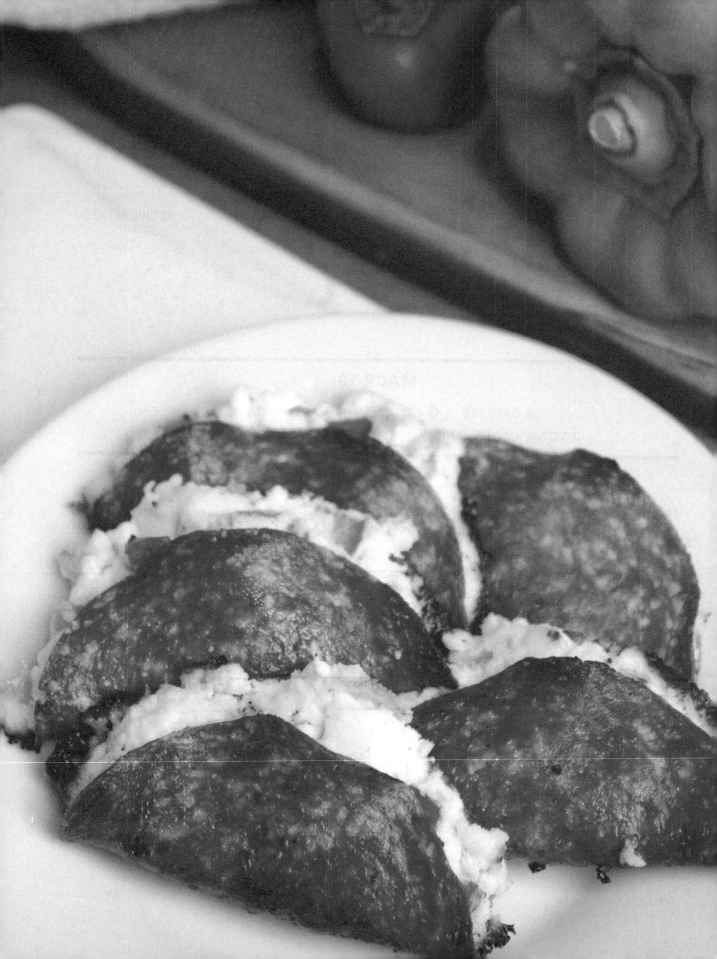

Salami Tacos

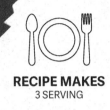

RECIPE MAKES
3 SERVING

MACROS

🔥 CAL: 321   ⬤ FAT: 40G   🫘 PROTEIN: 12G

🌾 TOTAL CARBS: 1G   🍃 FIBER: 0G   🌾 NET CARBS: 1G

INGREDIENTS

- 12 slices of salami
- 6 oz cream cheese
- 1/4 cup sliced bell peppers

INSTRUCTIONS

1. Combine all ingredients inside the salami and shape into tacos.

2. Bake on parchment paper at 400F for 15 minutes.

3. Take out, let cool & enjoy!

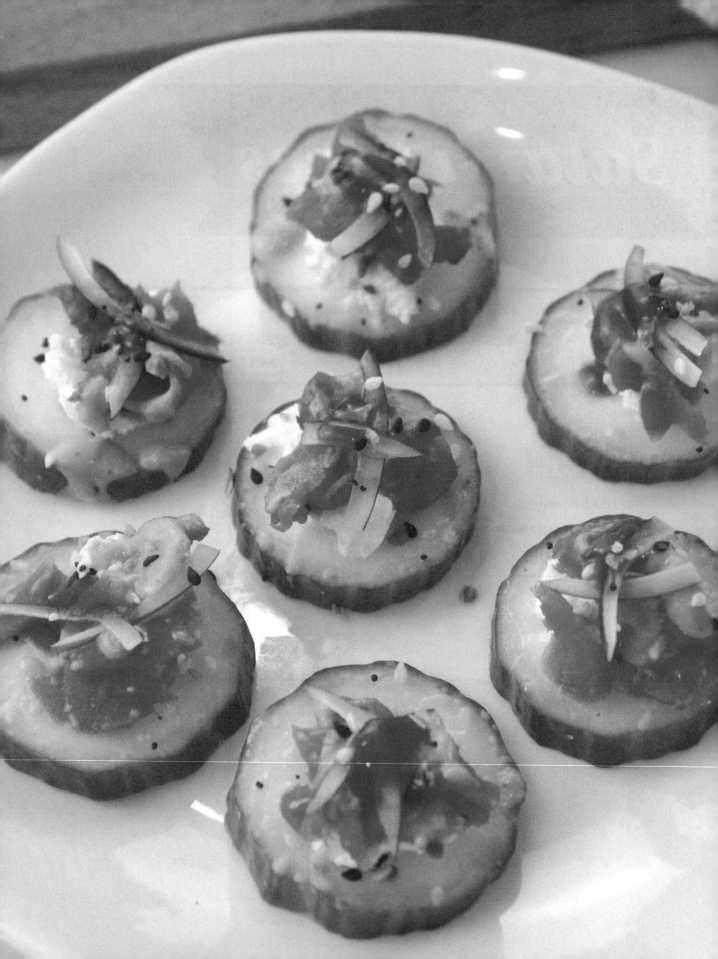

Smoked Salmon Bites

RECIPE MAKES
2 SERVING

MACROS

🔥 **CAL: 265**   🛢 **FAT: 18G**   🍳 **PROTEIN: 22G**

🌾 **TOTAL CARBS: 3G**   🍃 **FIBER: 1G**   🌾 **NET CARBS: 2G**

INGREDIENTS

- 1 medium cucumber
- 3 oz cream cheese
- 6 oz smoked salmon
- Salt

Optional:

- Everything bagel seasonings
- Sriracha mayo
- Thinly sliced red onion

INSTRUCTIONS

1. Slice & salt your cucumber.

2. Spread the cream cheese on each slice and add smoked salmon on top.

3. Top with your favorite ingredients & enjoy!

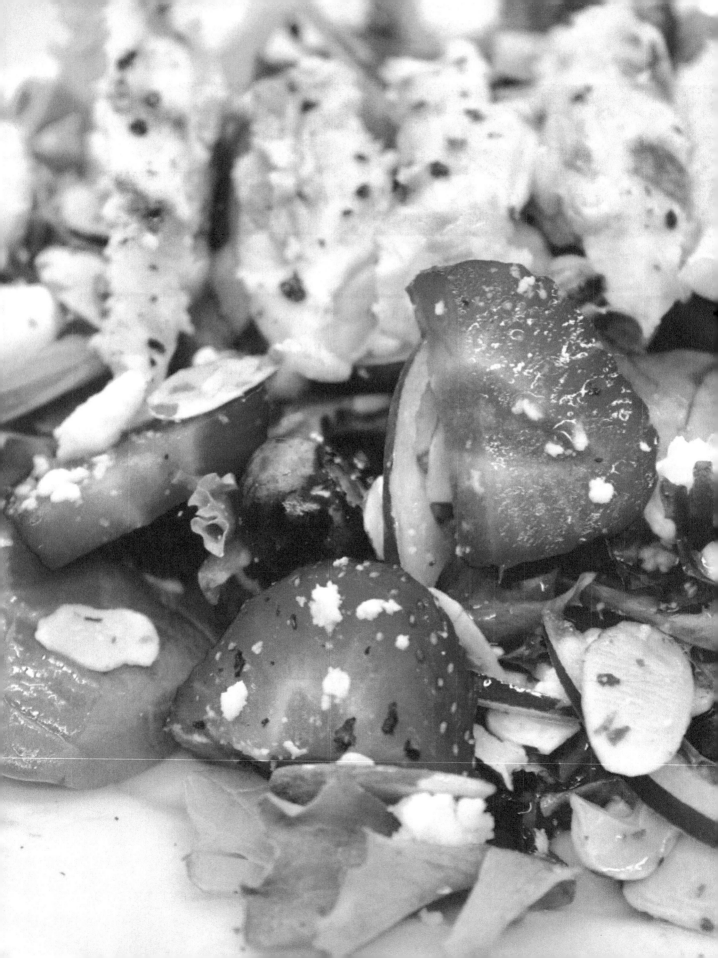

Strawberry Salad

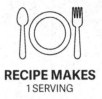

RECIPE MAKES
1 SERVING

MACROS

🔥 **CAL: 314**   🌢 **FAT: 18G**   🍳 **PROTEIN: 36G**

🌾 **TOTAL CARBS: 13G**   🍃 **FIBER: 32G**   🌾 **NET CARBS: 5.2G**

INGREDIENTS

- 1.5 cups spring salad mix
- 4 oz grilled chicken breast
- 1/4 cup crumbled goat cheese (or feta)
- 1/4 cup sliced strawberries
- 3 tbsp slivered almonds
- 3 tbsp blueberries
- 2 tbsp sliced red onions
- Dressing of your choice

INSTRUCTIONS

I. Mix all ingredients & enjoy!

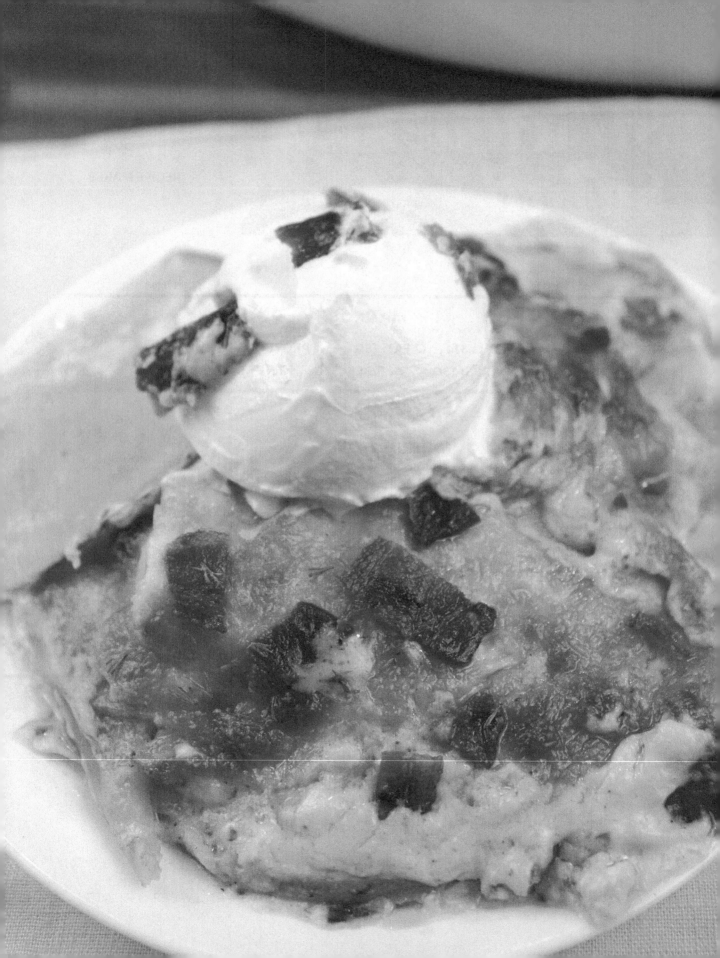

Scalloped Faux Tatoes

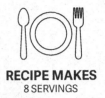

RECIPE MAKES
8 SERVINGS

MACROS

🔥 **CAL: 234**   🛢 **FAT: 20G**   **PROTEIN: 7G**

🌾 **TOTAL CARBS: 7G**   **FIBER: 1G**   🌾 **NET CARBS: 6G**

INGREDIENTS

- 3 cups rutabaga (thinly sliced)
- 1 cup shredded Colby Jack
- 1/2 cup heavy cream
- 1/2 cup chicken broth
- 1/2 cup shaved parmesan
- 2 tbsp olive oil
- 2 tbsp butter
- 2 tbsp cream cheese
- 1 tsp garlic powder
- 1 tsp onion powder
- 1/2 tsp salt
- 1/2 tsp pepper

Optional:

- Sour cream
- Bacon crumbles
- Herbs for garnish

INSTRUCTIONS

1. Preheat oven to 375F.

2. Slice rutabaga as thin as possible (I used a mandolin) and mix in a bowl with olive oil and seasonings. Add to a greased baking dish and set aside.

3. Combine the rest of your ingredients except the shredded colby jack in a saucepan over medium low and let simmer for 5 minutes.

4. Pour over the rutabaga slices, top with your Colby Jack & bake for 45 minutes.

5. Take out, top with bacon, sour cream & herbs.

6. Enjoy!

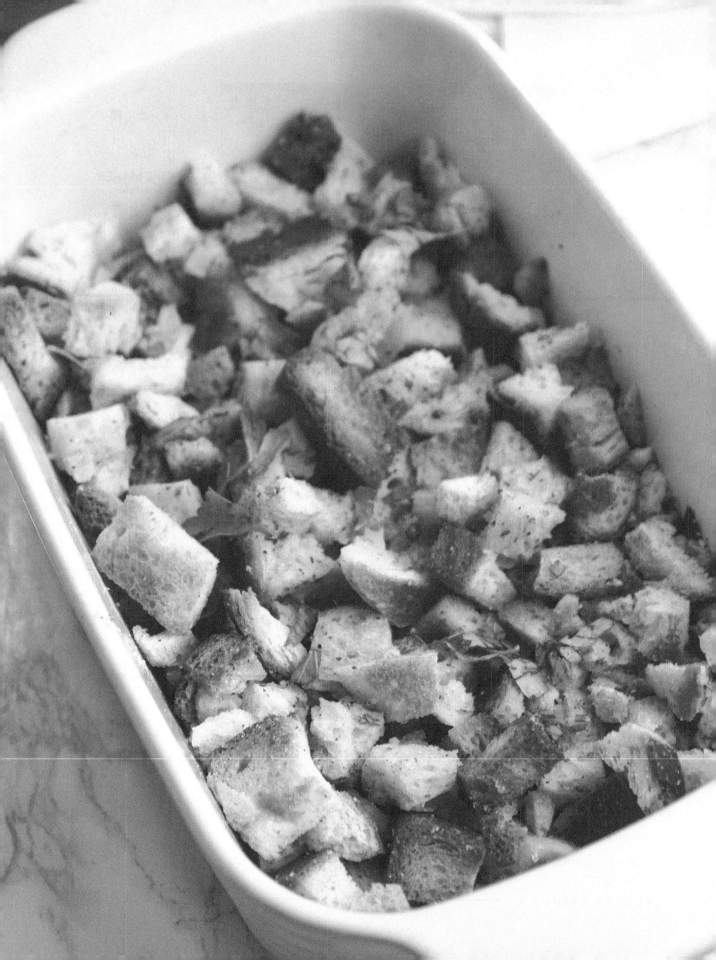

Stuffing

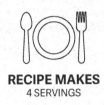

RECIPE MAKES
4 SERVINGS

MACROS

🔥 **CAL: 242**   🌢 **FAT: 23G**   ◖ **PROTEIN: 5G**

🌾 **TOTAL CARBS: 8G**   🍃 **FIBER: 4.4G**   🌾 **NET CARBS:3.6G**

INGREDIENTS

- 4 slices crumbled low carb bread
- 1/2 cup chicken broth
- 3 tbsp melted butter
- 3 tbsp olive oil
- 2 sticks of chopped celery
- 1/4 cup chopped green onions
- 1/2 tsp minced garlic
- 1/4 tsp dried oregano
- 1/4 tsp dried basil
- 1/4 tsp dried rosemary
- 1/4 tsp dried thyme
- 1/4 tsp sage
- Salt & pepper

INSTRUCTIONS

1. Preheat oven to 350F.
2. Coat bread crumbles with 2 tbsp olive oil and bake until lightly browned. (5 minutes)
3. Add vegetables & 1 tbsp olive oil to pan over medium heat for 1-2 minutes.
4. Combine everything in a large baking dish and cover.
5. Bake for 10 minutes, uncover and put back in for 5 more minutes.
6. Take out, let cool, & enjoy!

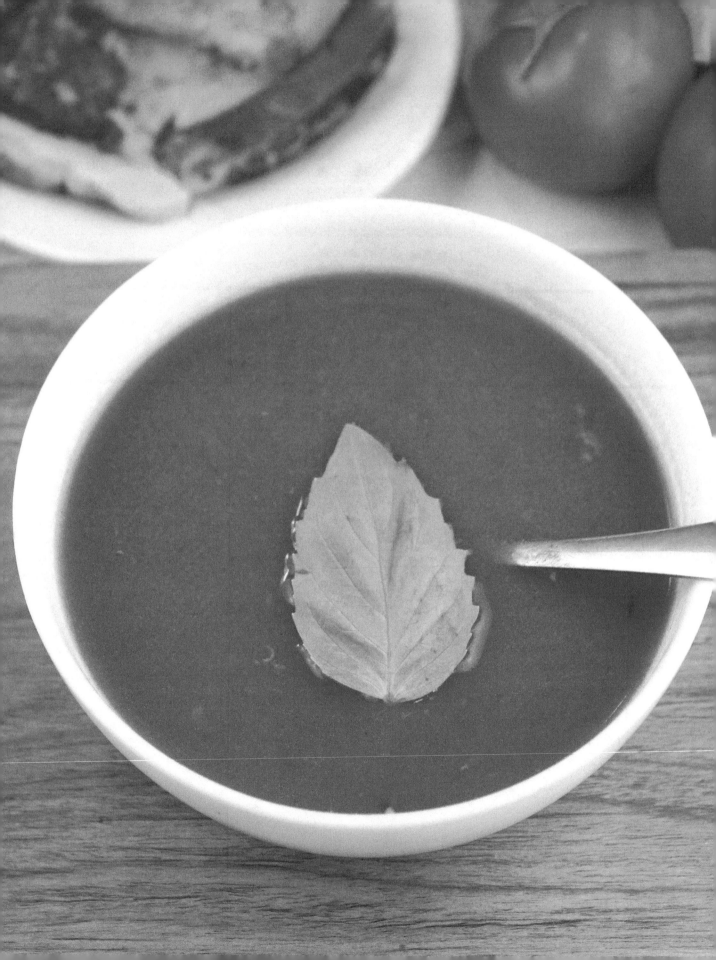

Tomato Soup

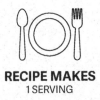

RECIPE MAKES
1 SERVING

MACROS

🔥 **CAL: 304**   💧 **FAT: 29G**   🥚 **PROTEIN: 3G**

🌾 **TOTAL CARBS: 8G**   🍃 **FIBER: 1G**   🌾 **NET CARBS: 7G**

INGREDIENTS

- 1/2 cup Raos marinara sauce
- 1/4 cup heavy cream

Optional:

- 1 tbsp sweetener

INSTRUCTIONS

1. Combine ingredients and microwave for 2 minutes.
2. Let cool & enjoy!

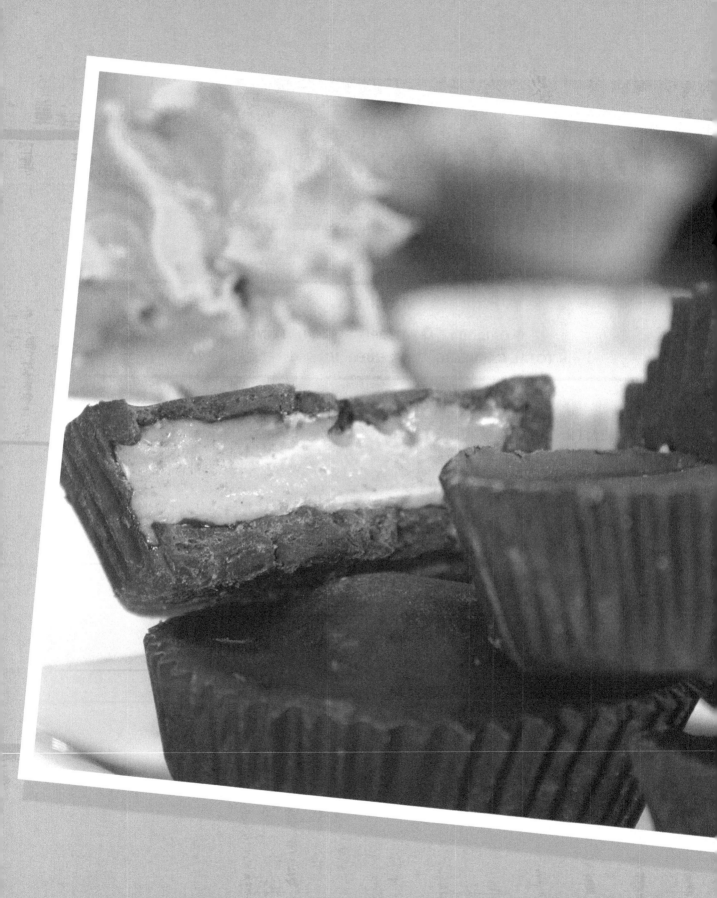

Sweet Treats

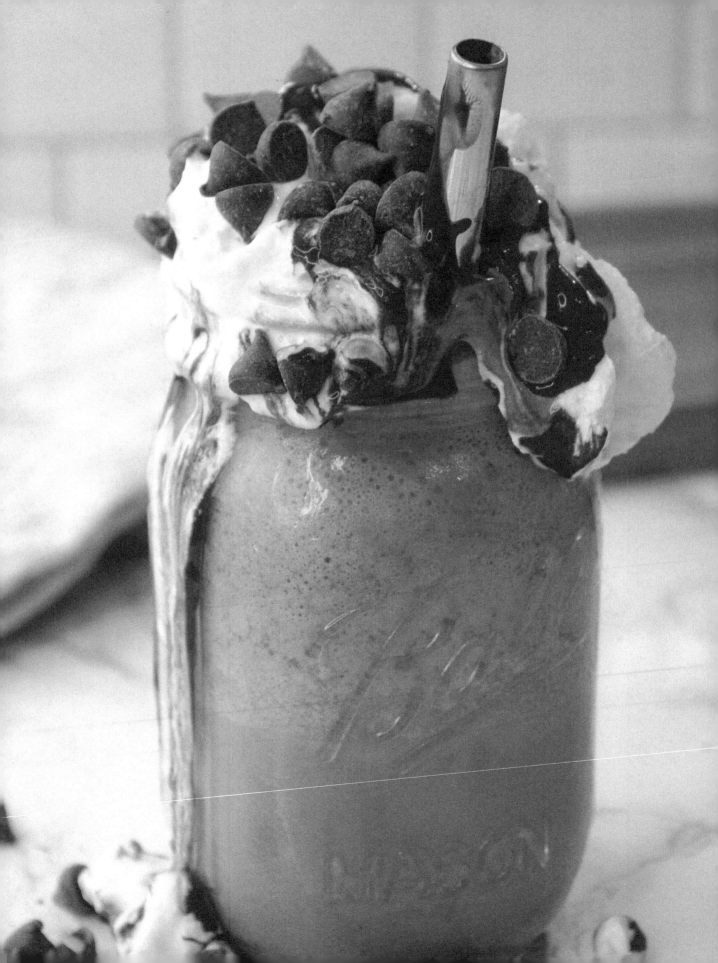

Chocolate chip Frappuccino

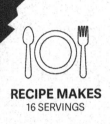

RECIPE MAKES
16 SERVINGS

MACROS

🔥 CAL: 118   🌢 FAT: 6G   🥚 PROTEIN: 12G

🌾 TOTAL CARBS: 9G   🍃 FIBER: 4G   🎁 SUGAR ALCOHOL: 3G   🌾 NET CARBS: 2G

INGREDIENTS

- 4 oz cold brew
- 4 oz caramel protein shake (or unsweetened milk of choice)
- 1/4 cup sugar free chocolate chips
- 1/2 cup ice

Toppings: (optional)

- Sugar free whipped cream
- Sugar free chocolate syrup

INSTRUCTIONS

1. Combine all ingredients & blend.

2. Run the blender 2-3 times to ensure the chocolate chips don't sink to the bottom.

3. Top with your optional ingredients & enjoy!

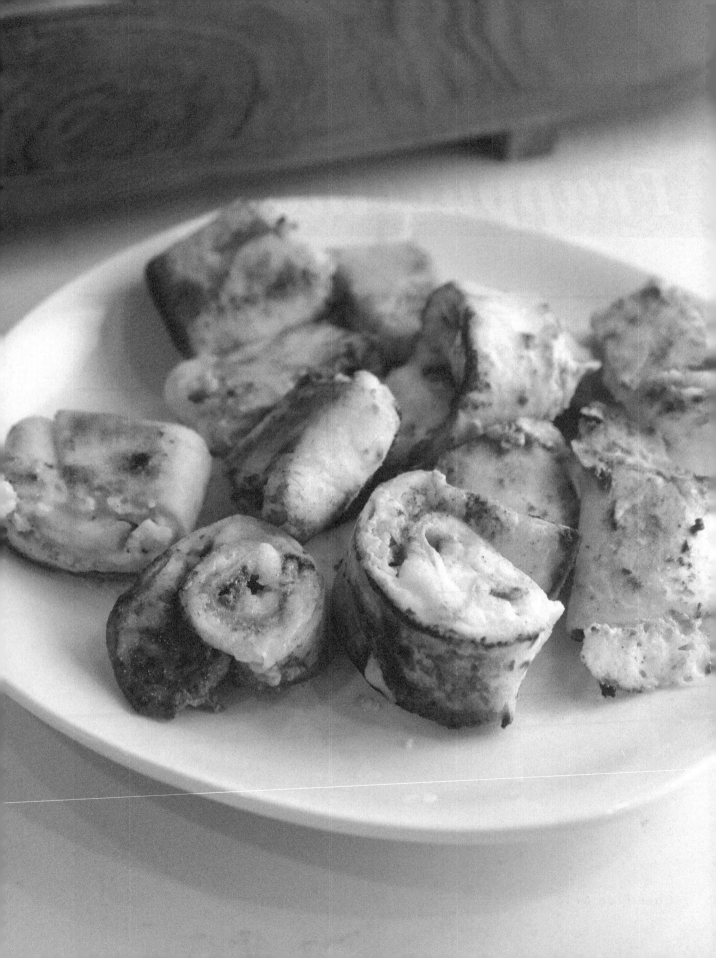

Cinnamon Roll Ups

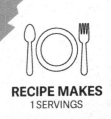

RECIPE MAKES
1 SERVINGS

MACROS

🔥 **CAL: 366** 🪔 **FAT: 34G** 🥚 **PROTEIN: 9G**

🌾 **TOTAL CARBS: 21G** 🍃 **FIBER: 15G** 🌾 **NET CARBS: 6G**

INGREDIENTS

- 1 low carb tortilla, 8 inch
- 2 oz cream cheese
- 1 tbsp butter
- 3 tbsp sweetener
- 1/2 tsp cinnamon

INSTRUCTIONS

1. Spread cream cheese, sweetener & cinnamon over your tortilla and roll up tightly.

2. Melt your butter and brush on the outside of the tortilla.

3. Air fry at 400F for 8-10 mins.

4. Slice into bite sized pieces & enjoy!

Notes:

Mix some powdered sweetener with milk or heavy cream and drizzle on top. I do about 3 tbsp sweetener per 3 tbsp of milk but you can adjust it to your desired thickness.

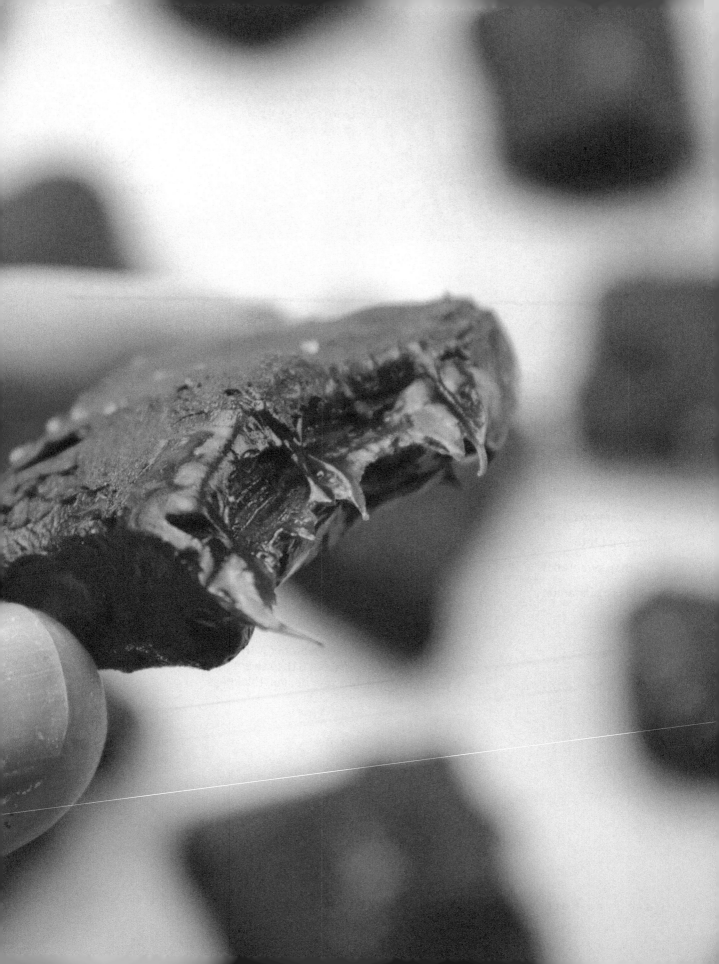

Caramel Chocolate

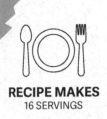

RECIPE MAKES
16 SERVINGS

MACROS

🔥 **CAL: 42**   🌢 **FAT: 3G**   🫘 **PROTEIN: 0.8G**

🌾 **TOTAL CARBS: 7.5G**   🍃 **FIBER: 3.8G**   🌾 **NET CARBS: 3.7G**

INGREDIENTS

- 1 cup low carb chocolate chips
- 1 tsp coconut oil
- 1/3 cup sugar free caramel sauce
- Sea salt

INSTRUCTIONS

1. Combine your chocolate chips with coconut oil in a bowl and microwave for 30 second intervals stirring between each one.

2. Drizzle the chocolate into 16 1"x1" molds, just enough to cover the bottom. Tap on the counter until it spreads evenly.

3. Freeze for 5 minutes and then layer your caramel sauce on top and place back in the freezer for 5 more minutes.

4. Reheat your bowl of chocolate in 15 second intervals and cover the caramel. Sprinkle it with sea salt and freeze for 10 minutes.

5. Store in the refrigerator and enjoy!

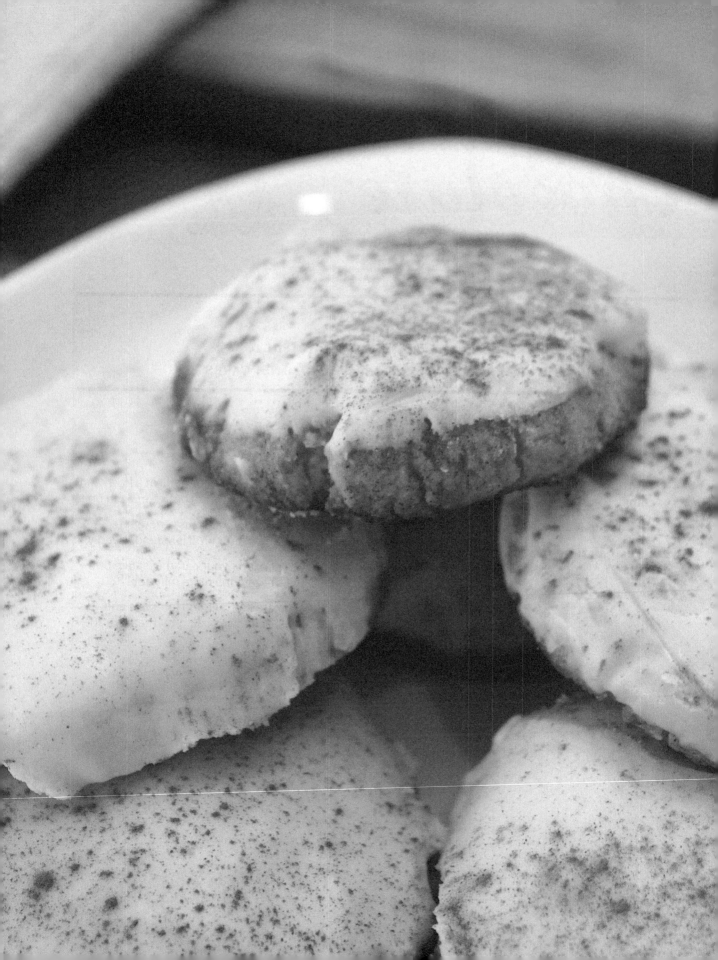

Cinnamon Toast Cookies

RECIPE MAKES
15 SERVINGS

MACROS

🔥 CAL: 177   🛢 FAT: 17G   🥑 PROTEIN: 3G

🌾 TOTAL CARBS: 4G   🍃 FIBER: 2G   🌾 NET CARBS: 2G

INGREDIENTS

For the cookies:

- 1/4 cup butter
- 3 oz cream cheese
- 1 large egg
- 1/2 cup powder sweetener
- 3 tbsp granular sweetener
- 1/2 tsp baking powder
- 1 tsp vanilla
- 2 tsp cinnamon
- 3/4 cup coconut flour (or 3 cups almond flour)
- Small pinch of salt

For the frosting:

- 8 oz cream cheese, softened
- 2 oz butter, softened
- 2/3 cup powdered sweetener
- 1 tbsp vanilla extract

INSTRUCTIONS

For the cookies:

1. Let butter and cream cheese soften.
2. Preheat the oven to 350F.
3. Mix butter and sweetener.
4. Add cream cheese, mix.
5. Add egg, baking powder, vanilla, 1/2 tsp cinnamon and salt, mix and add coconut flour and mix.
6. In a separate bowl mix granular sweetener and 1.5 tsp cinnamon.
7. Roll dough into 12-15 (2 tbsp) balls and then coat with the cinnamon mix.
8. Place balls on a parchment lined baking sheet and flatten. (Shape into cookies)
9. Bake for 15-20 minutes. Let cool 5 minutes, enjoy

For the frosting:

1. Combine all ingredients & mix well!

Notes
Swap the coconut flour for almond flour and get a much better texture.

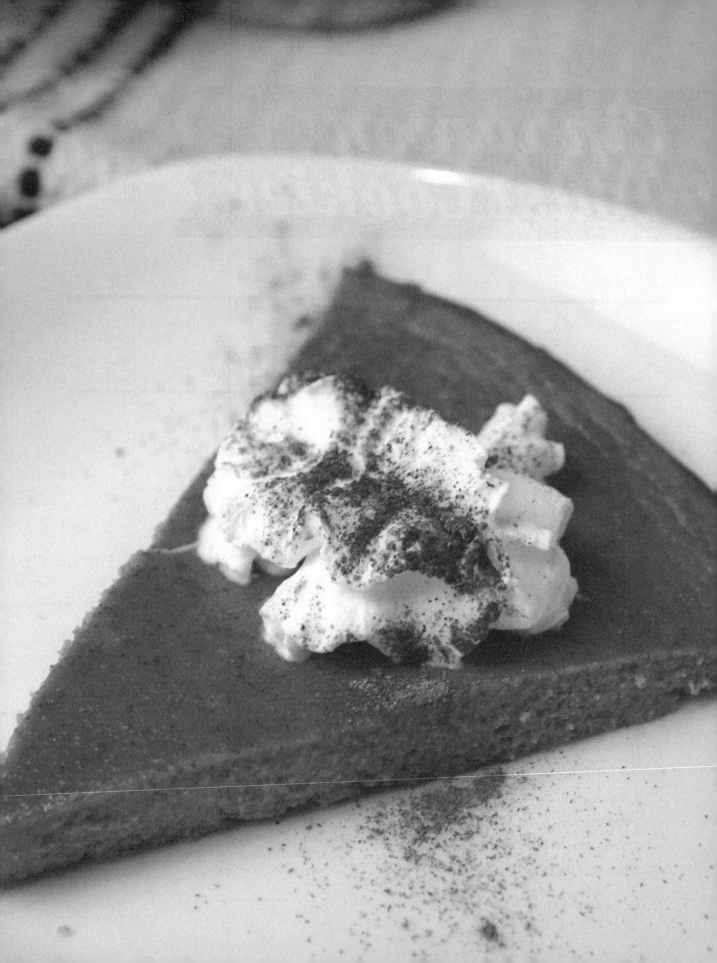

Crustless Pumpkin Pie

RECIPE MAKES
6 SERVINGS

MACROS

🔥 **CAL:** 122 　 🫗 **FAT:** 11G 　 **PROTEIN:** 4G

🌾 **TOTAL CARBS:** 5G 　 🍃 **FIBER:** 0.5G 　 🌾 **NET CARBS:** 4.5G

INGREDIENTS

- 1 can pumpkin purée
- 3 large eggs, beaten
- 3/4 cup heavy cream
- 3/4 cup sweetener
- 2 tsp pumpkin spice

INSTRUCTIONS

1. Preheat the oven to 350F.
2. Mix all ingredients & add to greased springform pan.
3. Bake for 30 minutes.
4. Take out, let cool, & enjoy!

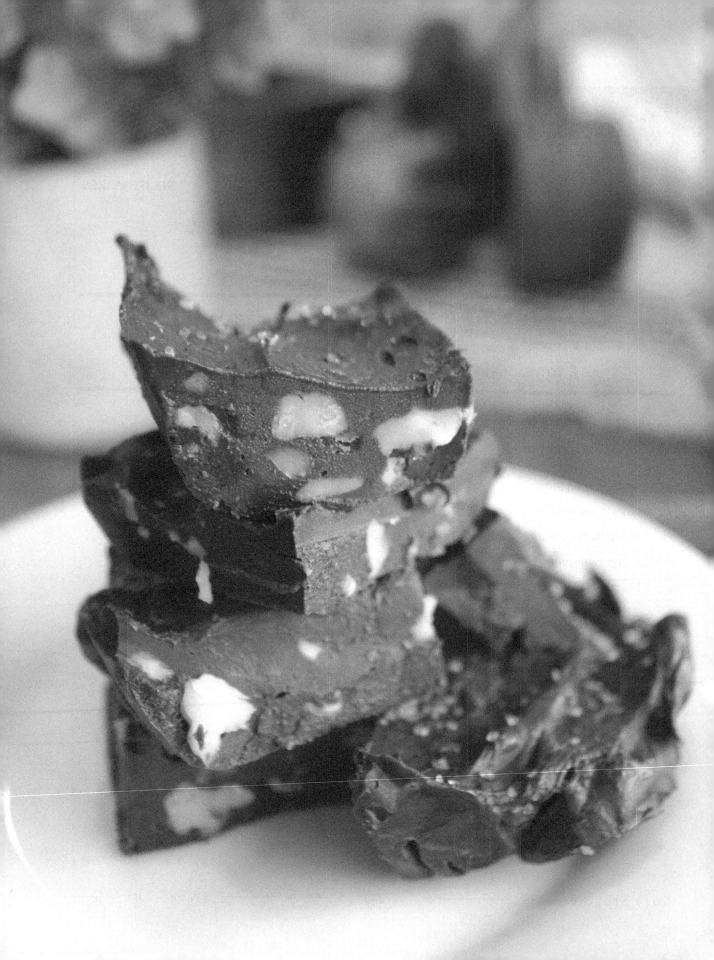

Chocolate Fudge

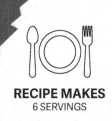

RECIPE MAKES
6 SERVINGS

MACROS

🔥 **CAL: 155**   ⬛ **FAT: 16G**   🫘 **PROTEIN: 0G**

🌾 **TOTAL CARBS: 5G**   🍃 **FIBER: 4G**   🌾 **NET CARBS: 1G**

INGREDIENTS

- 1/2 cup sugar free chocolate chips
- 4 tbsp butter
- 1/4 cup powdered sweetener
- 2 tbsp heavy cream

Optional:

- Nuts
- Dash of salt

INSTRUCTIONS

1. Microwave the butter and chocolate chips, stirring every 30 seconds until fully melted.

2. Combine remaining ingredients and add to a parchment lined dish.

3. Freeze until it hardens, chop it up & enjoy!

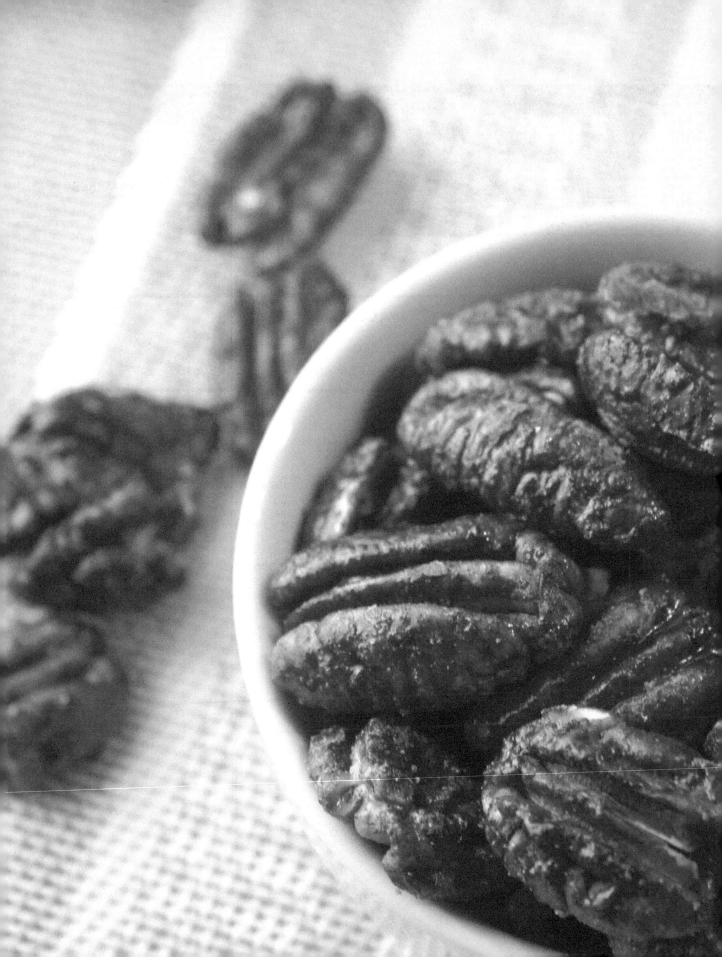

Candied Pecans

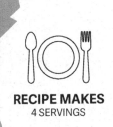

RECIPE MAKES
4 SERVINGS

MACROS

🔥 **CAL: 190** 🫗 **FAT: 20G** 🍖 **PROTEIN: 3G**

🌾 **TOTAL CARBS: 4G** 🍃 **FIBER: 3G** 🌾 **NET CARBS: 1G**

INGREDIENTS

- 1 cup pecans
- 3 tbsp keto brown sugar
- 1 tbsp water
- 1/2 tsp cinnamon
- 1/8 tsp cayenne (optional)

INSTRUCTIONS

1. Combine all ingredients except pecans in a bowl. Set aside.
2. Add pecans to a pan over medium heat until they become fragrant.
3. Add the mixture to the pecans and quickly remove from the heat stirring well to coat them.
4. Add to a parchment lined dish & let cool. (DO NOT TOUCH, THEY ARE SUPER HOT)

Note:

Keep an eye on the pecans, they can burn quickly.

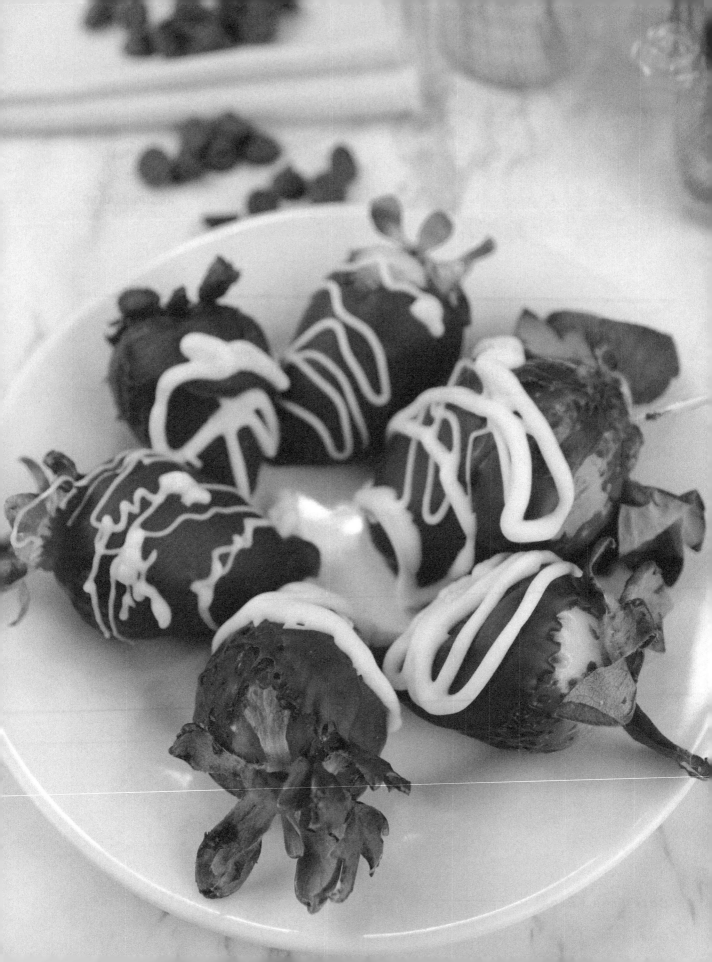

Chocolate Covered Strawberries

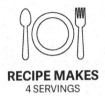

RECIPE MAKES
4 SERVINGS

MACROS

🔥 **CAL: 112**   🩸 **FAT: 7G**   🍖 **PROTEIN: 2G**

🌾 **TOTAL CARBS: 22G**   🍃 **FIBER: 12G**   🌾 **NET CARBS: 10G**

INGREDIENTS

- 1 lb strawberries
- 1/2 cup low carb chocolate chips

Optional:

- Low carb white chocolate chips

INSTRUCTIONS

1. Melt chocolate chips by microwaving in 20 second intervals and stirring until melty.

2. Dip your strawberries in the melted chocolate and add to a parchment lined dish.

3. Melt your white chocolate chips with the same method, drizzle on the chocolate covered strawberries.

4. Freeze for 20 minutes & enjoy!

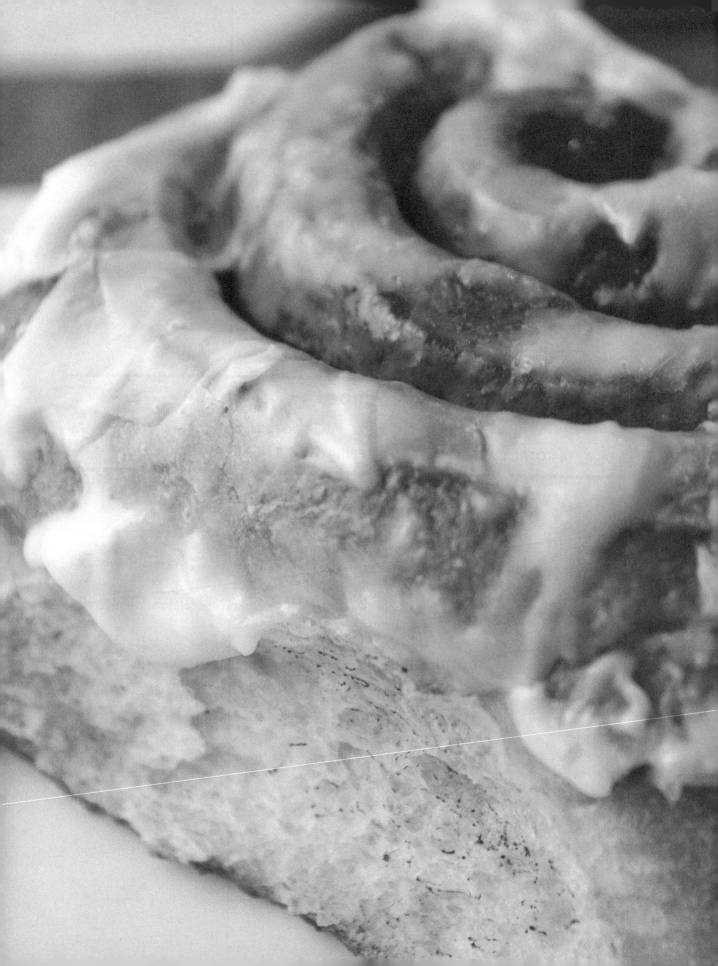

Cinnamon Rolls

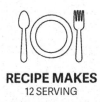

RECIPE MAKES
12 SERVING

MACROS

🔥 **CAL: 111**   💧 **FAT: 9G**   🥚 **PROTEIN: 5G**

🌾 **TOTAL CARBS: 2.2G**   🍃 **FIBER: 0.8G**   🌾 **NET CARBS: 1.4G**

INGREDIENTS

- 1.5 cups shredded mozzarella
- 3/4 cup almond flour
- 4 tbsp cream cheese, room temp
- 1 large egg
- 1/2 tsp baking powder
- 2 tbsp water
- 2 tbsp granular sweetener
- 2 tsp cinnamon
- 1 tbsp butter, room temp
- 2 tbsp powdered sweetener
- 1/2 tsp vanilla

INSTRUCTIONS

1. Preheat the oven to 360F.

2. Add mozzarella & 2 tbsp cream cheese to a bowl and microwave for 1 minute, stir and microwave for 1 more minute.

3. Mix together and set aside. In another bowl combine almond flour & baking powder and then add it to the mozarella mix along with one of the eggs.

4. Combine well and roll into a smooth ball. Divide into 6 balls of dough.

5. Form long rolls and flatten them between 2 sheets of greased parchment paper.

6. Bring the water to a boil and stir in the granular sweetener and cinnamon.

7. Spread the paste over each roll. Roll them into buns and cut them in half sideways.

8. Add to a non-stick baking dish and place in the oven for 20 minutes.

9. While baking, combine the remaining cream cheese, butter, powdered sweetener, & vanilla. Mix well until it forms a thick frosting. Take out the rolls, frost them while warm, & enjoy!

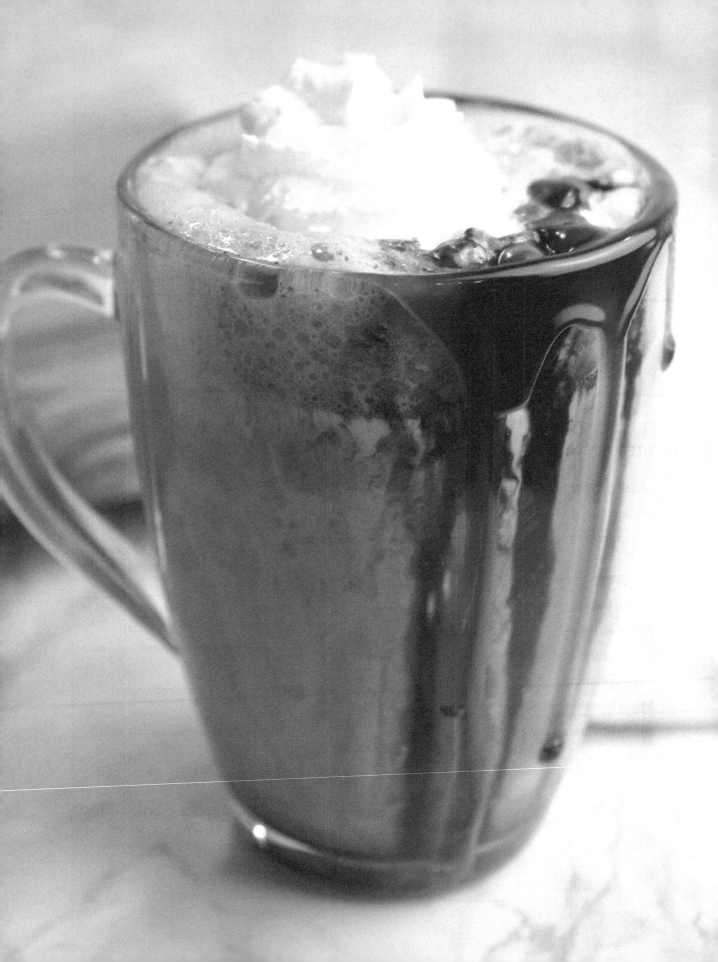

Hot Cocoa

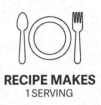

RECIPE MAKES
1 SERVING

MACROS

🔥 **CAL: 269**   🌢 **FAT: 27G**   🫘 **PROTEIN: 5G**

🌾 **TOTAL CARBS: 9G**   🍃 **FIBER: 4G**   🌾 **NET CARBS: 5G**

INGREDIENTS

- 12 oz unsweetened almond milk
- 4 oz heavy cream
- 3 tbsp sweetener
- 2 tbsp unsweetened cocoa powder

Optional:

- Sugar free whipped cream
- Sugar free chocolate syrup

INSTRUCTIONS

1. Add sauce pan to medium heat.
2. Pour in your almond milk and heavy cream until it begins to steam (5 minutes).
3. Whisk in the rest of your ingredients.
4. Pour into glass, add your favorite toppings & enjoy!

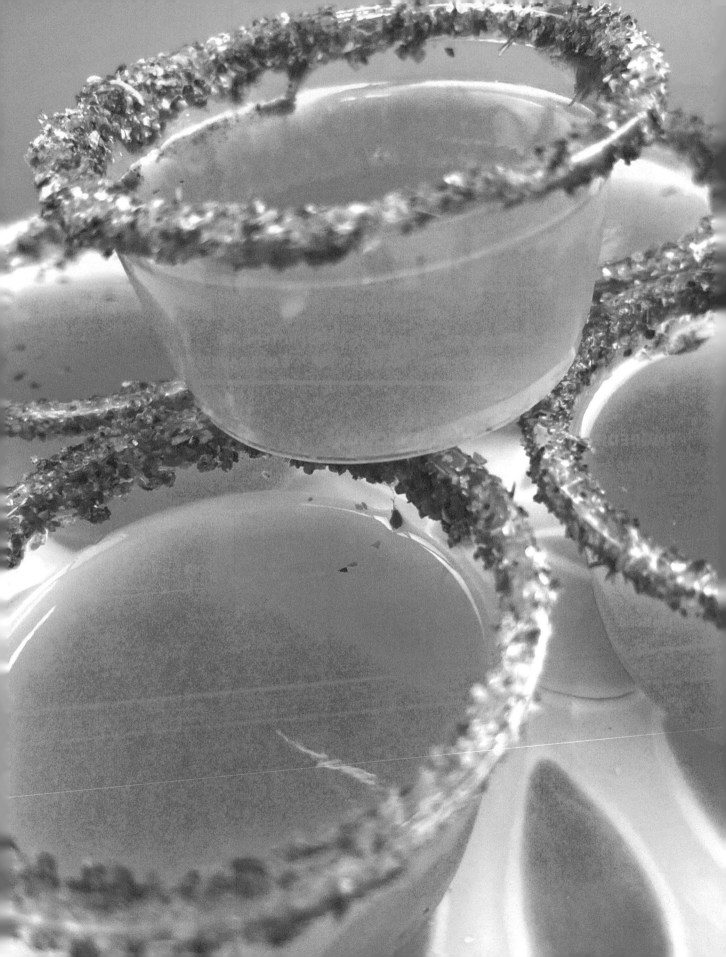

Jello Shots

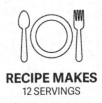

RECIPE MAKES
12 SERVINGS

MACROS

🔥 **CAL: 24**   🛢 **FAT: 0G**   🍳 **PROTEIN: 0G**

🌾 **TOTAL CARBS: 0.5G**   🐟 **FIBER: 0G**   🌾 **NET CARBS: 0.5G**

INGREDIENTS

- 1/2 cup tequila
- 1 tbsp unflavored gelatin
- 1/4 cup cold water
- 1/2 cup boiling water
- 1 tbsp allulose
- 1/3 cup fresh watermelon juice
- 1 lime, squeezed
- Chamoy
- Tajin

INSTRUCTIONS

I. In a medium bowl combine the gelatin and cold water, mix well and let rest for 2 minutes.

2. Add boiling water and sweetener, stir.

3. Add tequila, lime juice and watermelon juice and stir.

4. Dip the rim of your 12 shot containers in chamoy and then tajin. Place on a baking sheet for easy transport to the fridge.

5. Pour mixture into shot containers & refrigerate for at least 1 hour.

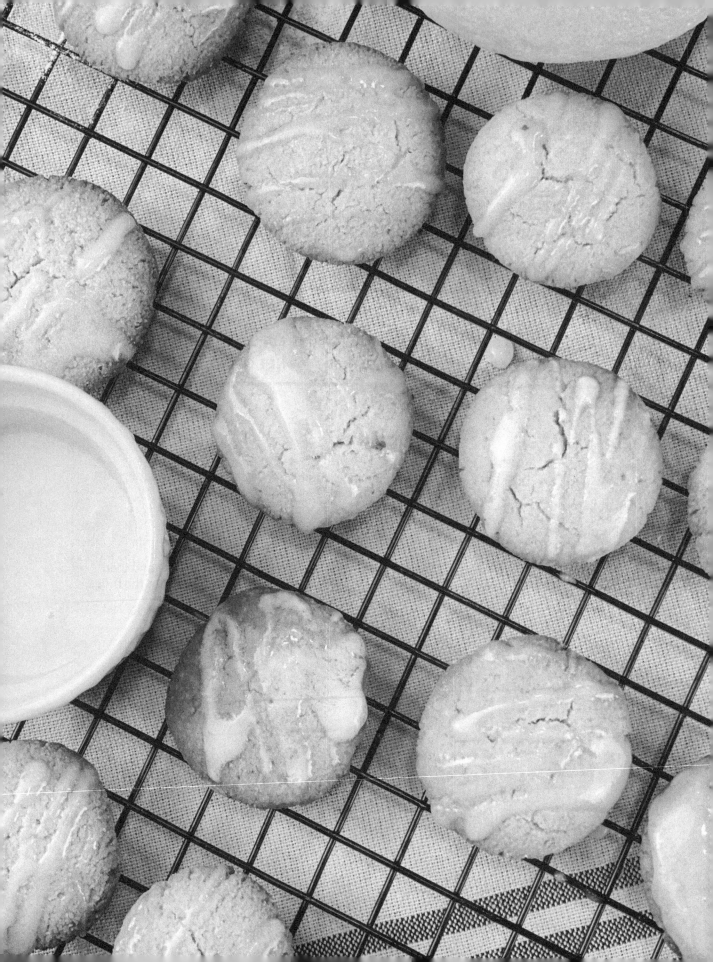

Lemon Cookies

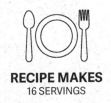

RECIPE MAKES
16 SERVINGS

MACROS

🔥 **CAL: 135**   🌢 **FAT: 13G**   🥩 **PROTEIN: 3G**

🌾 **TOTAL CARBS: 3G**   🍃 **FIBER: 1.5G**   🌾 **NET CARBS: 1.5G**

INGREDIENTS

- 2 cups almond flour
- 1 large egg
- 1/2 cup confectioners sweetener, swerve
- 1/2 tsp baking powder
- 1/2 cup butter
- 1 tsp vanilla
- 1/2 lemon, juiced

INSTRUCTIONS

1. Mix dry ingredients & set aside.
2. Mix wet ingredients & pour into the dry ingredients. Mix with a spoon until combined. Refrigerate for 30 minutes.
3. Preheat the oven to 300F.
4. Scoop 1 tbsp sized cookies on a parchment lined baking sheet with parchment paper.
5. Flatten the cookies & bake for 15-18 minutes.

Note:

For the frosting just mix 1/4 cup confectioners sweetener with the juice of 1/2 lemon & 1/2 tbsp heavy cream until it thickens.

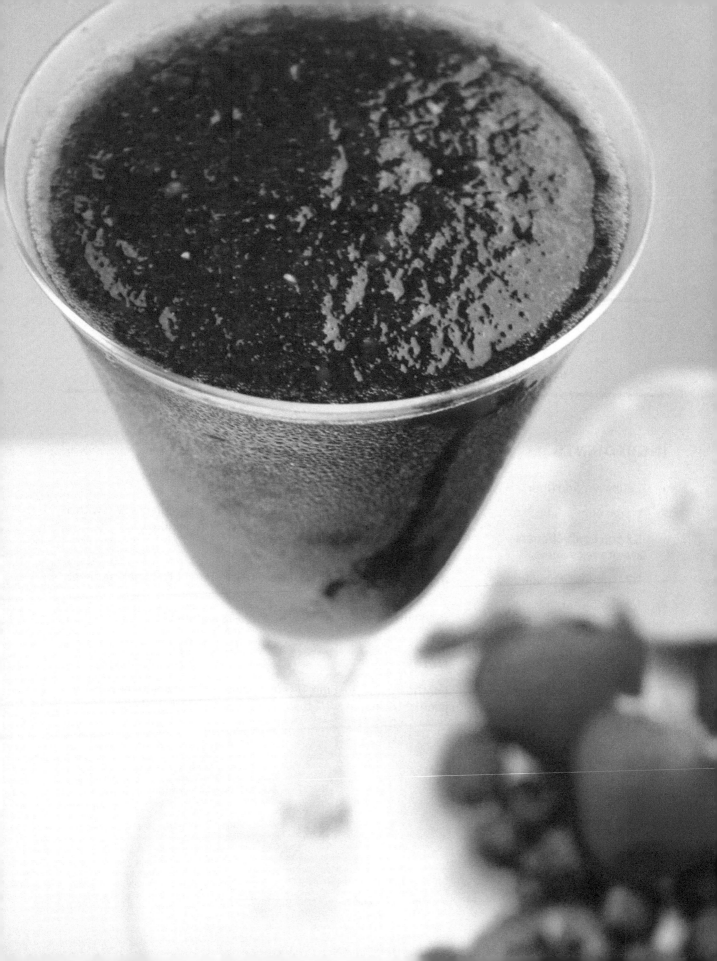

Lemon Berry Cocktail

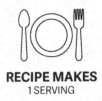

RECIPE MAKES
1 SERVING

MACROS

🔥 **CAL: 160** 🥑 **FAT: 0G** 🥚 **PROTEIN: 1G**

🌾 **TOTAL CARBS: 9G** 🍃 **FIBER:2G** 🌾 **NET CARBS: 7G**

INGREDIENTS

- 6 oz sugar free lemonade
- 1/4 cup frozen strawberries
- 1/4 cup frozen blueberries
- 1/4 cup ice
- 2 oz vodka

INSTRUCTIONS

1. Combine all ingredients and blend.
2. Pour into a glass, garnish, & enjoy!

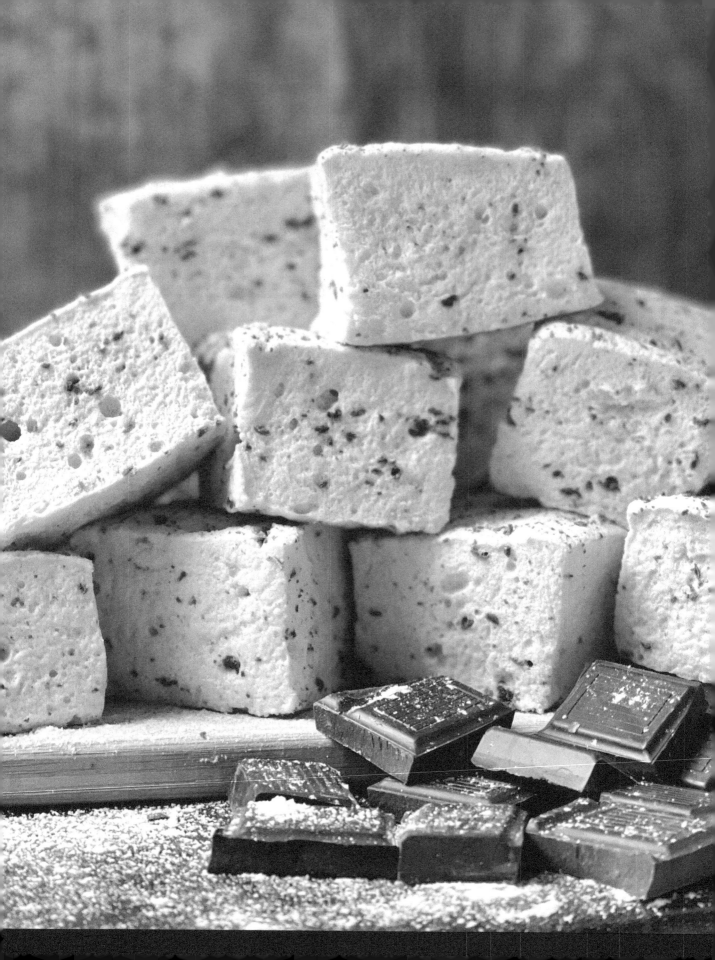

Marshmallows

RECIPE MAKES
1 SERVING

MACROS

💧 CAL: 32   🌢 FAT: 2G   🍳 PROTEIN: 1G

🌾 TOTAL CARBS: 3G   🍃 FIBER: 0G   🌾 NET CARBS: 0G

INGREDIENTS

- 1 cup granulated allulose
- 1/2 cup granulated brown sugar sweetener
- 3 tbsp unflavored gelatin powder
- 2 tsp vanilla extract
- 1.5 oz keto milk chocolate bar (grated)
- 1/2 tsp salt
- 1/2 cup water
- 2/3 cup water

INSTRUCTIONS

1. Line your pan with greased parchment paper and set aside.
2. In a large mixing bowl add the unflavored gelatin and 1/2 cup of water. Mix well and set aside for 10 minutes.
3. In a small sauce pan on medium high heat add 2/3 cup of water, allulose and brown sugar.
4. Combine and bring to a boil for 2 minutes.
5. Quickly add boiling sweetener to the gelatin while mixing with your mixer on low.
6. Once all the sweetener is added, mix on high for 15 minutes.
7. Halfway through mixing add salt. Once salt is mixed in, add the vanilla extract. Let it continue to mix until the 15 minutes is up.
8. After the 15 minutes is up, quickly fold in the grated chocolate with a spatula.
9. Pour marshmallow mixture into your pan and spread evenly.
10. Let sit for at least 8 hours before cutting.

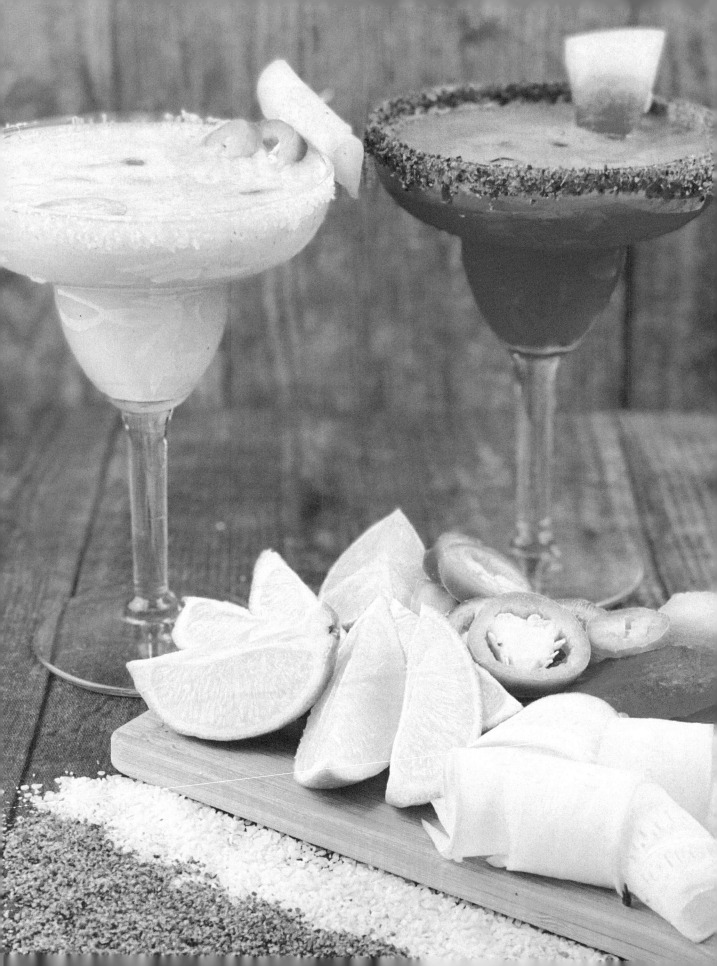

Margaritas

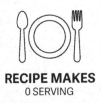

RECIPE MAKES
0 SERVING

MACROS

🔥 CAL: 140   🛢 FAT: 0G   🥚 PROTEIN: 0G

🌾 TOTAL CARBS: 4G   🍃 FIBER: 0G   🌾 NET CARBS: 0G

INGREDIENTS

- 3 cups ice
- 2 oz tequila
- 2 oz orange seltzer water
- 1 oz lime juice
- 2.5 tsp sweetener
- 1 tbsp coarse salt
- 2 lime wedges

INSTRUCTIONS

1. Fill a shaker halfway with ice.
2. Add tequila, lime juice, and sweetener to the shaker.
3. Shake as hard as you can for 15 seconds.
4. Dump your salt on a plate, rim the edge of your glass with a lime wedge. Press down the glass on the salt, fill the glass with the rest of your ice.
5. Pour the margarita into your glass, top with seltzer, and garnish with lime wedge.

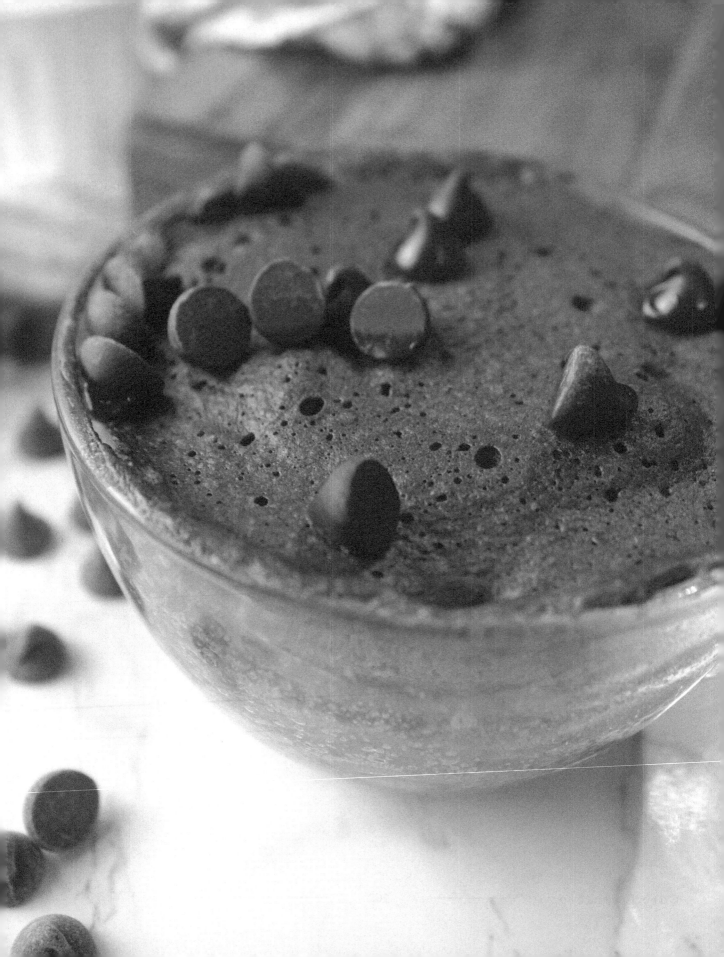

One Minute Brownie

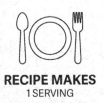

RECIPE MAKES
1 SERVING

MACROS

🔥 **CAL: 363**   ⬦ **FAT: 34G**   🥑 **PROTEIN: 7G**

🌾 **TOTAL CARBS: 12G**   🍃 **FIBER: 6G**   🌾 **NET CARBS: 6G**

INGREDIENTS

- 3 tbsp heavy cream
- 2 tbsp almond flour
- 1 tbsp unsweetened cocoa powder
- 1 tbsp sweetener
- 1 tbsp low carb chocolate chips
- 1 tbsp almond butter
- 1/8 tsp baking powder

INSTRUCTIONS

1. Mix dry ingredients and add to your mug.

2. Whisk together wet ingredients and stir into the mug.

3. Microwave for 1 minute, take out, let cool, & enjoy!

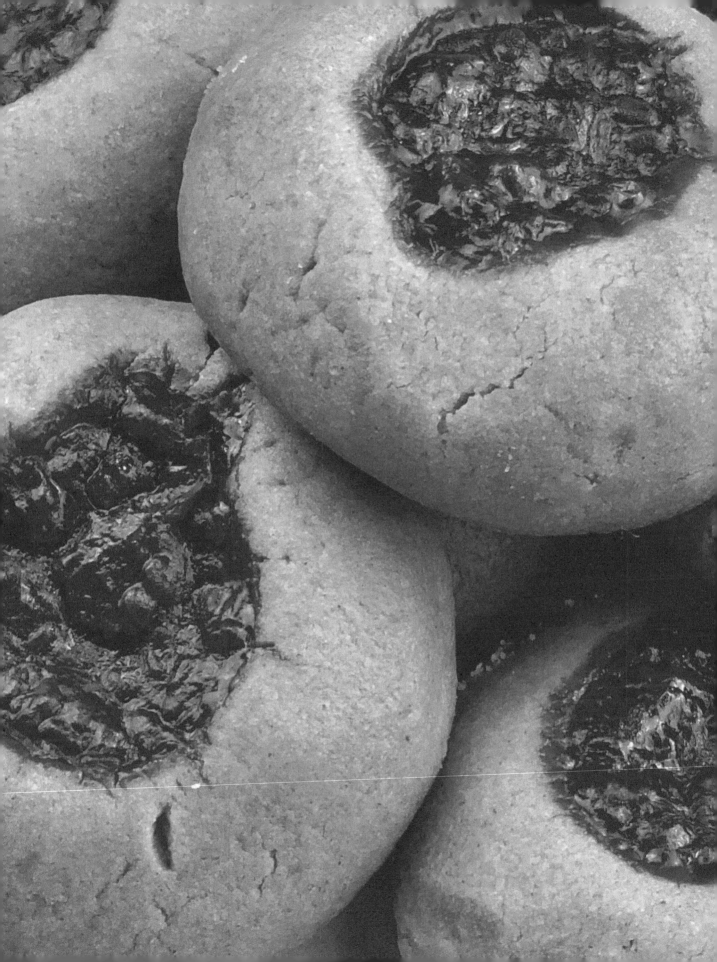

Peanut Butter & Jelly Cookies

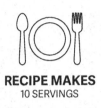

RECIPE MAKES
10 SERVINGS

MACROS

🔥 **CAL: 162**　　💧 **FAT: 13.4G**　　🍳 **PROTEIN: 7.1G**

🌾 **TOTAL CARBS: 6.3G**　　🍃 **FIBER: 2G**　　🌾 **NET CARBS: 4.3G**

INGREDIENTS

- 1 cup peanut butter
- 1 large egg
- 1/3 cup powder sweetener
- 1/4 cup strawberry jam (P. 287)

INSTRUCTIONS

1. Preheat the oven to 350F & line a baking sheet with parchment paper.

2. Mix all ingredients except jam.

3. Roll dough into 10 balls and add to the baking sheet.

4. Flatten the dough & press down with a tsp in the middle to make a thumbprint sized crater in the cookies.

5. Add 1 tsp jam to each crater and bake for 15 minutes. (Until golden brown)

6. Take out, let cool & enjoy!

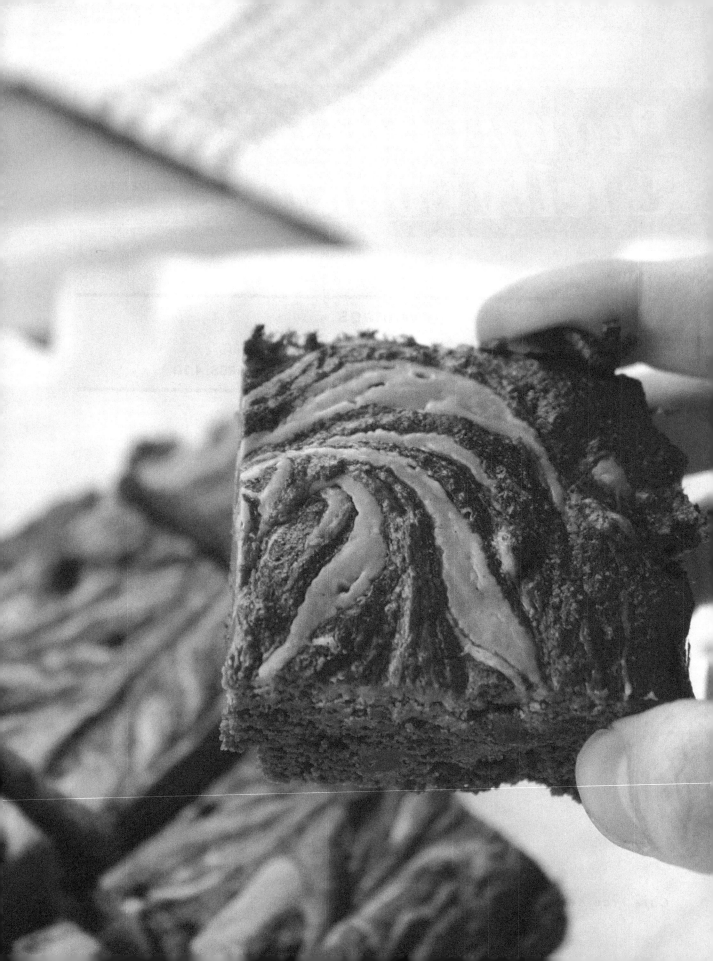

Peanut Butter Swirl Brownies

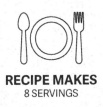

RECIPE MAKES
8 SERVINGS

MACROS

🔥 **CAL:** 252 　🥑 **FAT:** 7G 　🥚 **PROTEIN:** 23G

🌾 **TOTAL CARBS:** 10G 　🍃 **FIBER:** 6G 　🌾 **NET CARBS:** 4G

INGREDIENTS

- 1 cup almond flour
- 1/3 cup cocoa powder
- 1 tsp baking powder
- 1 cup sweetener
- 3 large eggs
- 1/3 cup butter, melted
- 1/2 cup sugar free chocolate chips
- 1/2 cup creamy peanut butter

INSTRUCTIONS

1. Preheat the oven to 350F.
2. Combine all ingredients, except for the chocolate chips & peanut butter
3. Fold in your chocolate chips and add to an 8x8 brownie pan.
4. Swirl in your peanut butter & bake for 35 minutes.
5. Take out, make sure a toothpick comes out clean & enjoy!

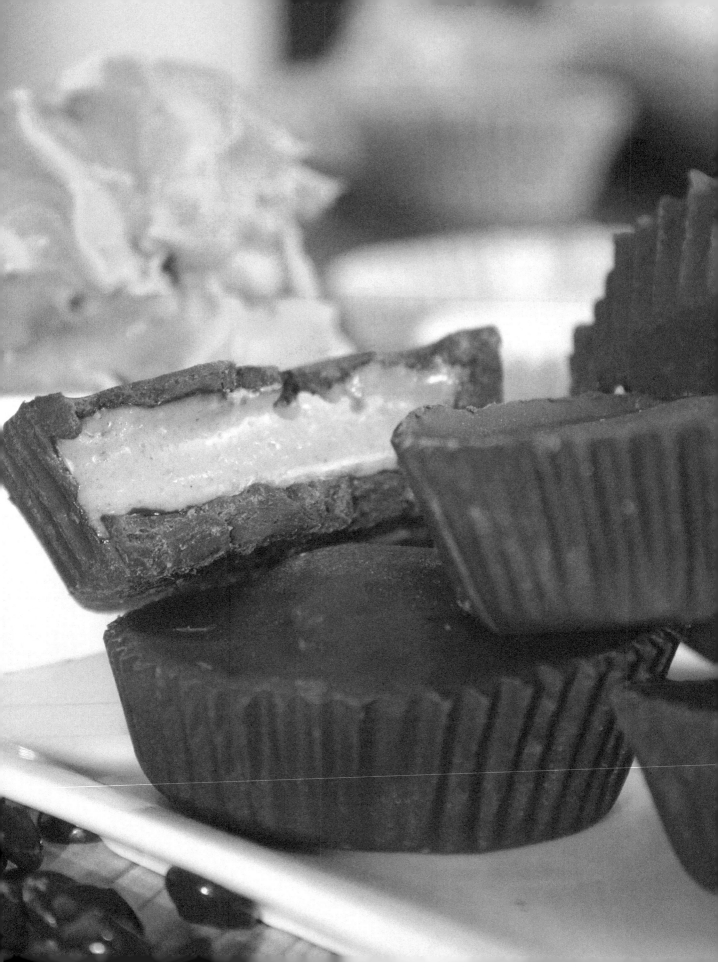

Peanut Butter Cups

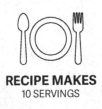

RECIPE MAKES
10 SERVINGS

MACROS

🔥 **CAL: 175**   🌢 **FAT: 15.6G**   🫘 **PROTEIN: 2.6G**

🌾 **TOTAL CARBS: 8.8G**   🍃 **FIBER: 6.6G**   🌾 **NET CARBS: 2.2G**

INGREDIENTS

Chocolate layer:

- 8 oz sugar free chocolate
- 2 tbsp sweetener (I used allulose)
- 1/4 cup coconut oil
- 1/2 tsp vanilla

Peanut butter filling:

- 3 tbsp peanut butter
- 1/2 tbsp coconut oil
- 1 tbsp powdered sweetener
- 1-2 tbsp almond flour (optional)
- 1/4 tsp vanilla
- 1 pinch salt

INSTRUCTIONS

1. Line a muffin tray with 10 nonstick cups.

2. Mix half of the ingredients for your chocolate layer, melt, and pour into the muffin cups. Freeze for 20 minutes.

3. Mix the filling ingredients, remove muffin tray from freezer and scoop the filling onto the chocolate in each muffin cup.

4. Melt the rest of your chocolate ingredients and cover the peanut butter in the muffin cups.

5. Freeze until the chocolate hardens and enjoy!

Notes:

1. When melting the chocolate I recommend microwaving for 20 second intervals stirring each time.

2. These don't store well at room temperature and will melt, so keep them in the freezer and eat immediately upon taking them out.

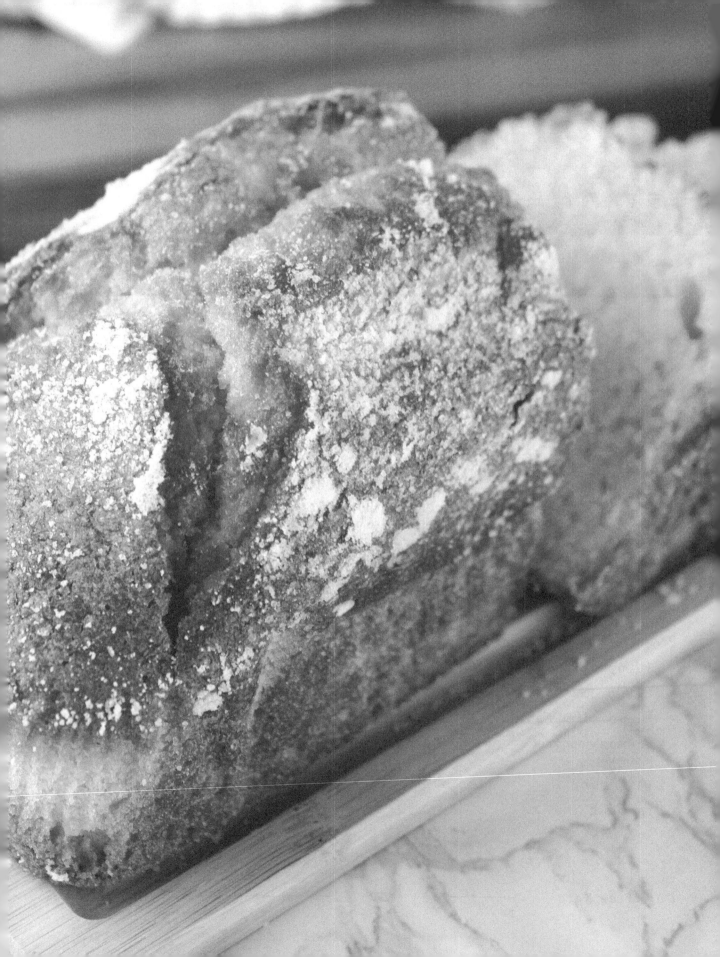

Pound Cake

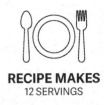

RECIPE MAKES
12 SERVINGS

MACROS

🔥 **CAL: 300**   💧 **FAT: 30G**   🥄 **PROTEIN: 7G**

🌾 **TOTAL CARBS: 6G**   🍃 **FIBER: 3G**   🌾 **NET CARBS: 3G**

INGREDIENTS

- 2.5 cups almond flour
- 1 cup butter
- 4 large eggs
- 2/3 cup allulose
- 1/2 tbsp baking powder
- 1/2 tbsp vanilla
- 1/2 tsp xanthan gum
- Salt

INSTRUCTIONS

1. Preheat the oven to 350F & line a loaf pan with parchment paper.
2. Beat the butter and allulose together until fluffy.
3. Mix in the eggs one at a time. Continue beating for 30 seconds between each one.
4. Slowly mix in your dry ingredients on a low mix setting.
5. Pour into your loaf pan and bake for 25 minutes.
6. Cover with foil and put back in for another 25-30 minutes. (Until a toothpick comes out clean).
7. Let the bread rest for 30 minutes before slicing.
8. Enjoy!

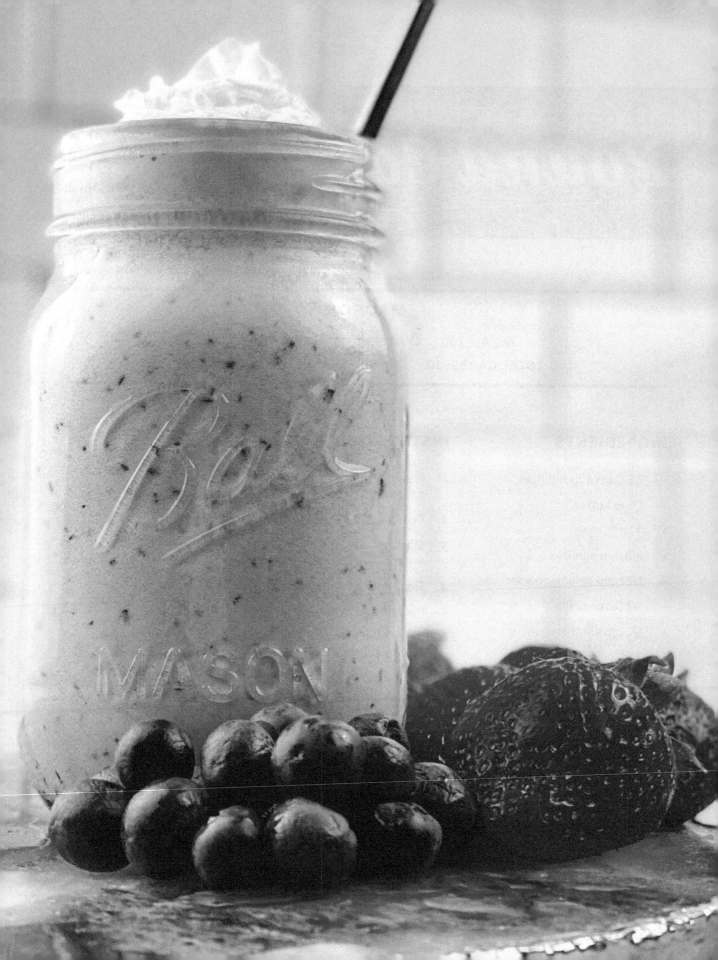

Protein Smoothie

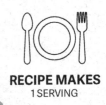

RECIPE MAKES
1 SERVING

MACROS

🔥 **CAL: 202**   🌢 **FAT: 3G**   🥟 **PROTEIN: 27G**

🌾 **TOTAL CARBS: 26G**   🍃 **FIBER: 17.5G**   🌾 **NET CARBS: 8.5G**

INGREDIENTS

- 4 frozen strawberries
- 1/4 cup frozen blueberries
- 1 cup unsweetened almond milk
- 1 scoop of unflavored protein powder
- 1 Tbsp of choc zero SF caramel syrup

INSTRUCTIONS

I. Combine all ingredients in blender, blend on high, pour into a glass & enjoy!

Note:

Replace the blueberries with raspberries to make this lower in carbs.

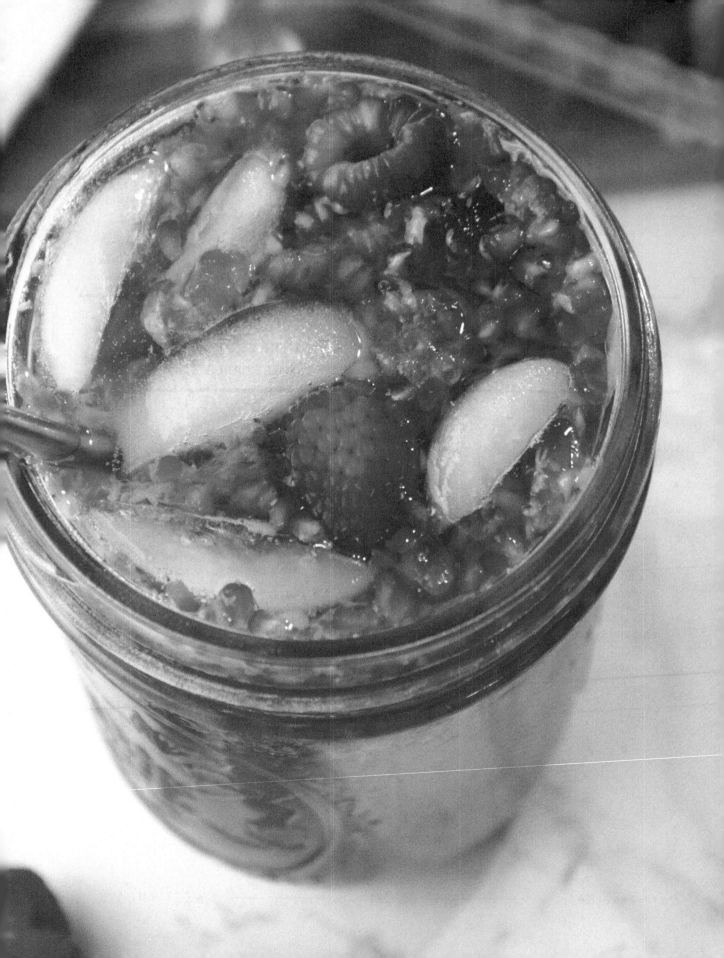

Raspberry Cocktail

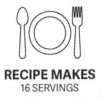

RECIPE MAKES
16 SERVINGS

MACROS

🔥 **CAL: 144**   🥑 **FAT: 0G**   🍳 **PROTEIN: 0G**

🌾 **TOTAL CARBS: 4G**   🌿 **FIBER: 2G**   🌾 **NET CARBS: 2G**

INGREDIENTS

- 1/4 cup fresh raspberries
- 2 shots of tequila
- 6 oz Sprite Zero

INSTRUCTIONS

I. Muddle together the raspberries & tequila.

2. Stir in your sprite with ice & enjoy!

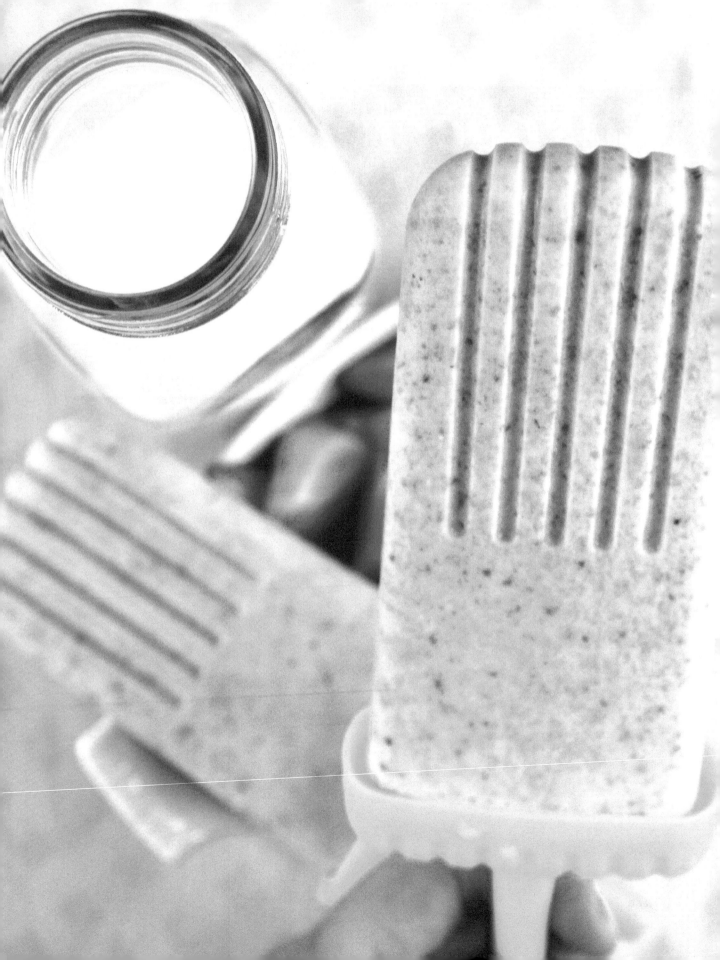

Strawberry Creamsicles

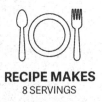

RECIPE MAKES
8 SERVINGS

MACROS

🔥 **CAL: 222**   🥑 **FAT: 0.5G**   🫘 **PROTEIN: 24.5G**

🌾 **TOTAL CARBS: 4.3G**   🍃 **FIBER: 1G**   🌾 **NET CARBS: 3.3G**

INGREDIENTS

- 1 lb strawberries
- 2 cups heavy cream
- 1 cup unsweetened almond milk
- 1/3 cup sweetener
- 2 tsp vanilla

INSTRUCTIONS

1. Blend all ingredients.
2. Add to 8 popsicle molds.
3. Freeze for 6 hours. (until solid)
4. Run under warm water before eating.

Note:

You can use 1 cup of heavy cream and 2 cups of almond milk to lower the calories.

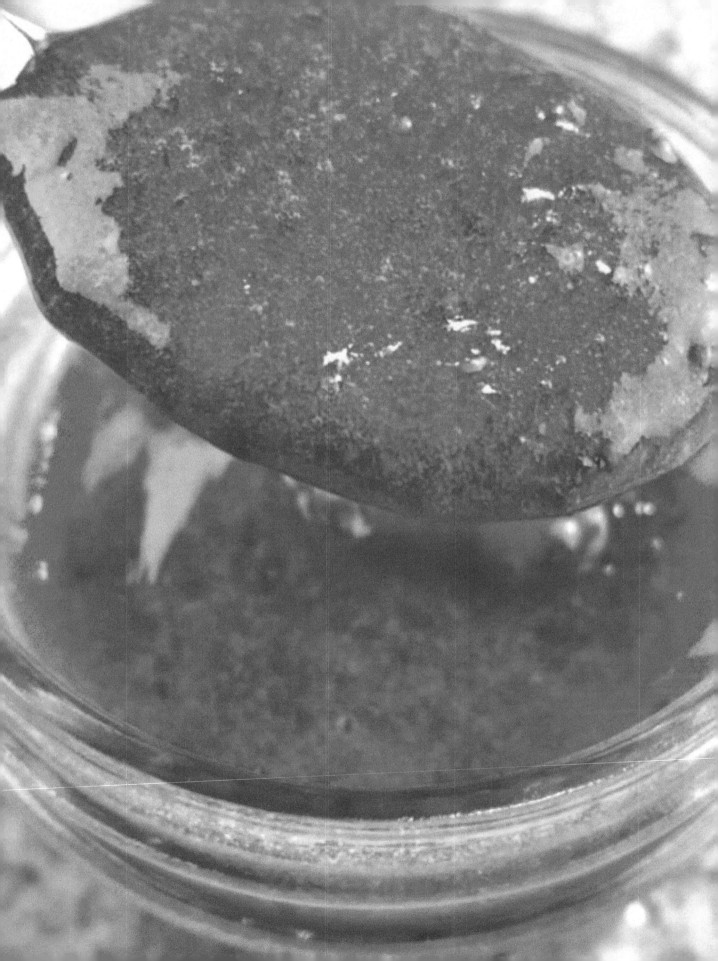

Strawberry Jam

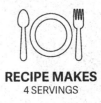

RECIPE MAKES
4 SERVINGS

MACROS

🔥 **CAL: 36**   💧 **FAT: 0.2G**   🌀 **PROTEIN: 0.8G**

🌾 **TOTAL CARBS: 8.7G**   🍃 **FIBER: 2.5G**   🌾 **NET CARBS: 6.2G**

INGREDIENTS

- 1 lb sliced strawberries
- 1.5 cups sweetener
- 2 tbsp lemon juice

INSTRUCTIONS

1. Add your strawberries to a sauce pan on medium heat and mix in the sweetener.

2. Stir until you bring the strawberries to a boil.

3. Once boiling add your lemon juice.

4. Let boil for another 15 minutes / until jam reaches 220F.

5. Stir often so the jam doesn't burn.

6. Pour into a jar and let cool. Once it's no longer hot, let chill in the fridge & enjoy!

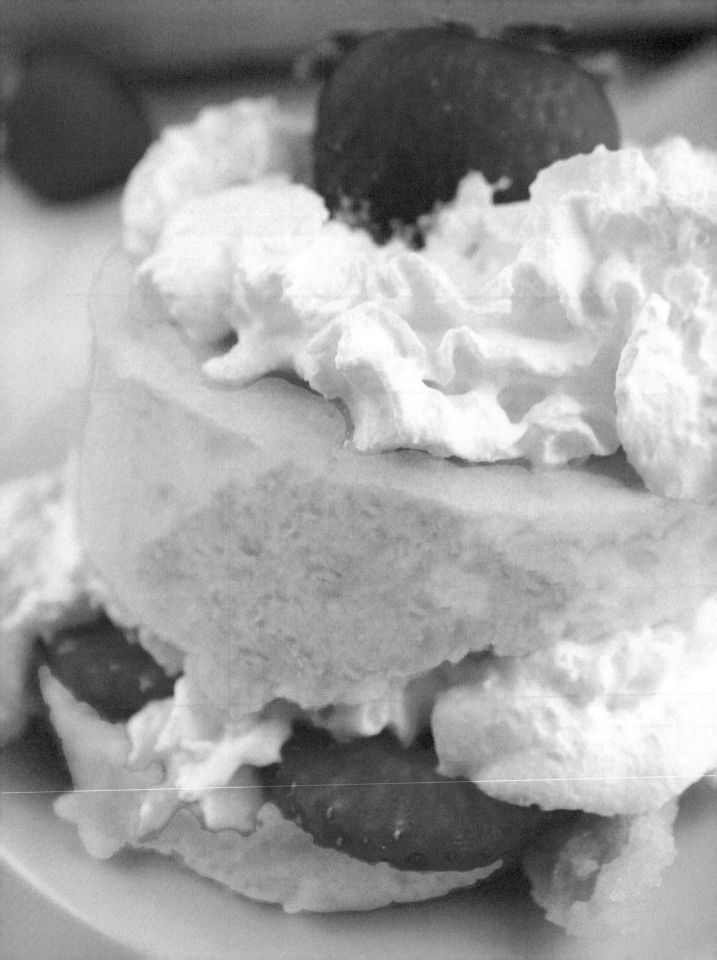

Strawberry Shortcake

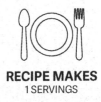

RECIPE MAKES
1 SERVINGS

MACROS

🔥 **CAL: 614**   🌢 **FAT: 53G**   🥄 **PROTEIN: 16G**

🌾 **TOTAL CARBS: 16G**   🍃 **FIBER: 8G**   🌾 **NET CARBS: 8G**

INGREDIENTS

- 6 tbsp almond flour
- 2 tbsp sweetener
- 2 tbsp butter
- 1 large egg
- 1/2 tsp baking powder
- 1/2 tsp vanilla extract
- 1/2 cup sliced strawberries
- 4 tbsp sugar free whipped cream

INSTRUCTIONS

1. Melt the butter in a mug.

2. Add the rest of your ingredients except the whipped cream & strawberries.

3. Mix well & microwave 90 seconds or until firm.

4. Dump out on plate, cut in half, add your strawberries & whipped cream to each layer and enjoy!

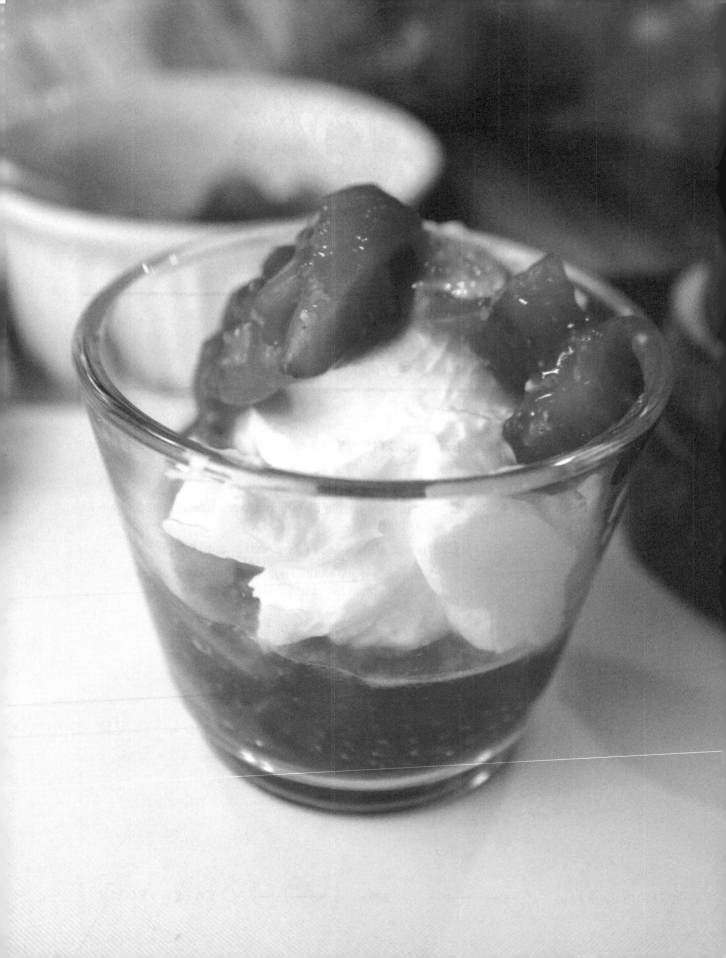

Strawberry Cheesecake Cups

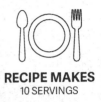

RECIPE MAKES
10 SERVINGS

MACROS

🔥 **CAL: 107**   🫗 **FAT: 11G**   🍖 **PROTEIN: 1G**

🌾 **TOTAL CARBS: 2G**   🍃 **FIBER: 0.3G**   🌾 **NET CARBS: 1.7G**

INGREDIENTS

- 1 cup heavy cream
- 1 cup strawberries, sliced
- 1 tbsp sweetener
- 4 oz cream cheese
- 1/4 cup powdered sweetener
- 1 tbsp sweetener
- 1 tbsp lemon juice

INSTRUCTIONS

1. Add heavy cream to a mixing bowl and beat on high with a hand mixer until it starts to thicken.

2. Add your cream cheese and powdered sweetener, continue beating.

3. When stiff, add 1/2 tbsp lemon juice & beat until firm.

4. Mix your strawberries with the rest of your lemon juice & granular sweetener, mash together.

5. In 4 jars add 1 tbsp strawberry mixture & 2 tbsp cream mixture to each.

6. Drizzle the remaining strawberry mixture on top.

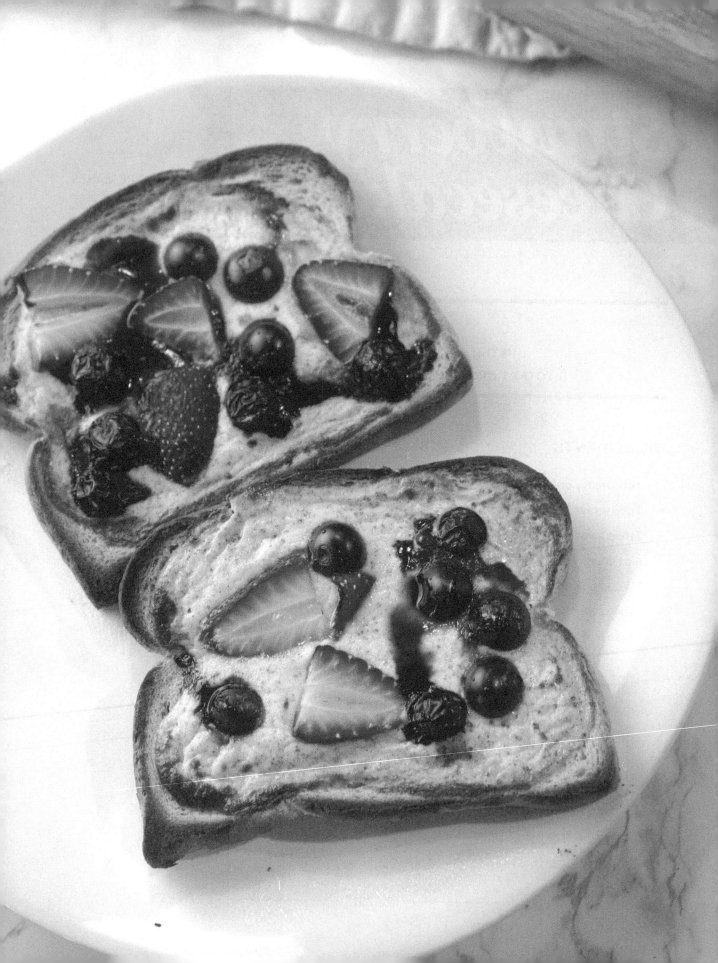

Yogurt Toast

RECIPE MAKES
4 SERVINGS

MACROS

🔥 CAL: 148   🌢 FAT: 6G   🥚 PROTEIN: 10G

🌾 TOTAL CARBS: 25G   🍃 FIBER: 18.4G   🌾 NET CARBS: 6.6G

INGREDIENTS

- 4 slices of low carb bread
- 1 cup two good vanilla yogurt
- 1 large egg
- 4 tbsp sugar free syrup
- 1 tbsp monk fruit (or sweetener of choice)
- 1 tsp cinnamon
- 1/4 cup fresh strawberries
- 1/4 cup fresh blueberries

INSTRUCTIONS

1. Preheat the oven to 400F.
2. Combine egg with yogurt, 3 tbsp syrup, & 3/4 tsp cinnamon.
3. Add your bread to a parchment lined baking sheet & spread on the yogurt mix.
4. Top with berries & sprinkle your sweetener on.
5. Bake for 15 minutes.
6. Take out, drizzle the remaining syrup & sprinkle cinnamon on top.
7. Enjoy!

DISCLAIMER:

The information in this book is not medical advice and should not be used to encourage any lifestyle changes without the reader first consulting a physician. The publisher and author are not responsible for any health or allergy issues that may require medical attention and are not liable for any damages or negative consequences from any actions taken by anyone who reads or follows the information in this book.

For permission requests, contact the author:
irick@ketosnackz.com

CREDITS:

Book Design
Puang Fikar (@puangfikar)

Proofing
Sandy Butler, Steffanie Moyers

Recipe development
Ana Olivero

Made in the USA
Las Vegas, NV
10 November 2023